Praise for
Cosmetic Breast Surgery

"This is one of the most informative and best organized books on breast surgery that I have ever seen. It contains a tremendous wealth of information and important examples that will be of benefit to every breast surgery patient. Every woman contemplating breast surgery should start with this resource."

—ANNETTE BRICCA, founder of www.BreastHealthOnline.org

"Dr. Freund, an accomplished plastic surgeon, has written an exceptionally informative book for women contemplating breast surgery. In a clear and factual tone, he skillfully explains the multitude of surgical options and their risks and rewards. His sensitive advice helps potential patients not only understand themselves better, but also make intelligent and informed choices for their anticipated surgery."

—NICHOLAS TABBAL, MD, FACS

Robert M. Freund, MD, FACS
with Alexander Van Dyne

Cosmetic Breast Surgery

A Complete Guide to

Making the Right Decision

—from A to Double D

MARLOWE & COMPANY
NEW YORK

COSMETIC BREAST SURGERY
A Complete Guide to Making the Right Decision—from A to Double D
Copyright © 2004 by Robert M. Freund
Illustrations by Lauren Raio

Published by
Marlowe & Company
An Imprint of Avalon Publishing Group Incorporated
245 West 17th Street • 11th Floor
New York, NY 10011-5300

Library of Congress Cataloging-in-Publication Data

Freund, Robert M., 1961-
    Cosmetic breast surgery : a complete guide to making
the right decision—from A to double D / Robert M.
Freund, with Alexander Van Dyne.
        p. cm.
    Includes index.
    ISBN 1-56924-455-3
    1. Breast—Surgery—Popular works. I. Van Dyne, Alex.
II. Title.

RD539.8.F73 2004
618.1'90592—dc22

                                    2004042636

            9 8 7 6 5 4 3 2

Designed by Pauline Neuwirth, Neuwirth & Associates, Inc.

Printed in the United States of America
Distributed by Publishers Group West

Cosmetic breast surgery has undergone major advances in the recent past. The shapes are better, the scars are smaller. But what is right for you? This book is dedicated to every woman interested in cosmetic breast surgery searching for fair and balanced information.

Contents

Introduction

BREAST SURGERY IS now entering its second century of existence, and for good reason. It is one of the most widely chosen types of surgery performed today, for both cosmetic and reconstructive purposes.

The first efforts at breast surgery began near the turn of the last century. The Industrial Revolution was just getting into full swing, and a doctor in Vienna, Robert Gersuny, had an idea for increasing the breast size of his female patients. He was almost certainly not the first person to come up with this idea (or at least fantasize about it), but he is credited as the first doctor to attempt a surgical procedure to make it happen. His technique involved injecting paraffin into the breast tissue. Although his efforts were not successful, the groundwork was set.

More than a hundred years later, medical science has, thankfully, come a long way. Millions of surgical procedures have been successfully completed and a multitude of lives have been positively changed. Now you are considering cosmetic breast surgery. You have many questions, or at least I hope you do, because it is a big decision. Cosmetic surgery is *surgery*. There are many things that you need to consider before taking this big step.

There are social issues: What will your friends and family think about you doing this? Perhaps your boyfriend, husband, or lover has strong opinions on the subject. There are health issues: What are the risks associated with the surgery you are considering? There are many aesthetic issues: What kind of surgery do you want? Do you want to be bigger or smaller? How much bigger or smaller? Or maybe you want a lift or reconstruction after a mastectomy. Is one breast larger or smaller than you desire? Where will you have scarring and how noticeable will it be? Perhaps you have not had children yet and are worried about breast-feeding. These are just some of the many important questions you should ask yourself.

During this time you should absorb all of the information you can. Find a surgeon you can trust and talk about all aspects of the surgical procedure you are considering. You might have to meet with your surgeon several times before you are satisfied that you really know exactly what you want from this process—and exactly what your surgeon can and can't provide for you. There is a tremendous amount of information about breast surgery available on the Internet, but unfortunately there is also a tremendous amount of disinformation, so don't trust everything you read online. If you have friends who have undergone the same procedure, ask questions. They are excellent sources of information. Become an informed patient!

There is so much information that you should gather before having cosmetic breast surgery that really you should read a book on the subject. As a dedicated plastic surgeon, I searched my local bookstore for an appropriate book that I could recommend to my patients. Surprisingly, I couldn't find one, despite the fact that 650,000 women undergo cosmetic breast surgery every year. So I decided to write my own.

MY EXPERIENCE WITH COSMETIC BREAST SURGERY

AT THE TIME of my training as a plastic surgery resident at New York University Medical Center ten years ago, success in cosmetic breast surgery was defined by the idea that any improvement was good, no matter how small. The techniques for breast reductions had remained the same for twenty years and were limited by boxy shapes, nipples that pointed toward the sky, and excessive scarring. Techniques for sagging breasts were even more disheartening. Patients were either relegated to getting implants much larger than they desired in order to take out the droop, or excess skin was removed with resultant scars and limited durability. I often told patients that they would complain about the scars for the first year, and when they got tired of that complaint they would start complaining that the droop had returned.

During my training and early on in my private practice in New York and at the prestigious Manhattan Eye, Ear and Throat Hospital, I asked colleagues if there was a better way to perform these surgeries in order to improve the aesthetic outcomes, but was met with discouraging responses, like "This is the way it's done," or "Patients won't tolerate any new techniques." But change was in the air. On a trip to the Caribbean while researching the forms of many young shapely women, I came to an epiphany that there had to be a better way—a way to make large breasts smaller and shapelier, a way to lift sagging breasts with durability and no excessive scars.

First, I set out to study the new techniques of surgeons in Belgium and Brazil. Doctors from these countries were experimenting with techniques that did the things I was looking to accomplish. My own application of these techniques confirmed the quantum improvements possible, and I eventually developed the teardrop augmentation mastopexy—a technique to moderately enlarge and lift sagging breasts, giving them natural teardrop breast contours.

More than a thousand cosmetic breast procedures later, I find little use for the techniques that were touted in my training as "the way it is done." The techniques from Belgium have become the basis for an abundance of new procedures that limit scars and maximize the natural breast shape, and are widely available. The popularity of the Brazilian technique is lagging behind because of the steep learning curve, but the improvements are no less amazing.

In the ten years since my residency, I have seen many patients who were unaware of the new cosmetic breast surgery procedures. Often these patients, without an understanding of the new treatments and their benefits, had previously seen another surgeon and were coming to me for a second opinion. This brings me back to the reason for this book. It is a guide women can utilize for a fair and balanced description of cosmetic surgery and all the available techniques. You may not be a candidate for the newest or coolest technique, but by reading this book you will no longer be in the dark.

WHAT YOU WILL FIND IN THIS BOOK

THIS BOOK IS not an advertisement for cosmetic breast surgery. In an effort to be fair and balanced, I begin by discussing if surgery is right for you. Any surgery is a serious decision. But when the surgery is done for purely cosmetic reasons, you must be certain that the benefits outweigh the risks. Subsequently, I carefully outline the risks and benefits as well as the factors that go into deciding what will be the perfect breasts for you. Other factors discussed include how to pick your surgeon and whether or not breast-feeding will be jeopardized as a result of your surgery. The terms you see in **boldface** are defined in the glossary in the back of the book. The illustrations throughout the text and before-and-after photos in the middle of the book are there to help you better visualize the procedures I discuss.

I also present in depth all the important factors and considerations necessary for you to decide if breast enlargement is right for you. Silicone implants have unfairly gotten a bad name as a result of several greedy trial lawyers and their ability to feed public hysteria. Things may be changing, and Chapter Eight, "The Silicone Implant Controversy," will help you to understand the past, present, and future of silicone gel implants.

Breast augmentation is only a fraction of the 650,000 cosmetic breast surgeries performed each year. Although it is the procedure most talked about in the media, there are other breast issues that warrant discussion. The chapters on breast reduction and breast lifts (Chapter Nine and Chapter Ten, respectively) discuss topics near and dear to my heart. In view of the recent explosion of new techniques, these chapters are more important now than ever before.

As a cosmetic breast surgeon, I often have woman walk into my office with asymmetrical breasts who are burdened by the feeling that they are all alone and without hope. Chapter Eleven, "Correcting Mismatched Breasts" clearly describes this very common problem and the many tailored techniques available to create a happy, self-confident patient. Chapters Twelve and Thirteen discuss how to correct previous breast surgeries and the complications of breast reconstructions after cancer surgery.

The important final two chapters in this book are for patients, friends, relatives, and parents. Why are breasts all the rage? What in our society has made large breasts so important to a girl's self-confidence? In Chapter Fourteen, Dr. Jennifer N. Duffy, PhD, a world-renowned expert in psychology of the breast, discusses why breasts are important and gives advice on how to sort reasonable breast concerns from unreasonable ones. It is not always easy for a surgeon to identify patients who are having surgery for all the wrong reasons. Dr. Duffy's chapter will shed light on this most important topic.

Finally, in Chapter Fifteen, I discuss teens and breast surgery. More and more, I have teenagers walking into my office requesting breast surgery with their reluctant parents in tow. What is the parent to do? This chapter will enlighten the wary and concerned parents and friends of these teen patients. It will hopefully aid them in making the correct decisions for their daughter or friend.

If you are considering cosmetic breast surgery, this book is for you. It is also for your family and friends. Cosmetic breast surgery is personal and your situation is unique. This book is your ally and tool in helping you make the best decisions you can.

While I am a doctor and not a writer per se, the stories and information presented in this book had to be told. This is a user-friendly guide, written by an expert on breast surgery, designed to educate and empower women considering cosmetic breast surgery, as well as their friends, family, and significant others. It is my hope that, after reading this book, you will be more informed of your specific problems and considerations regarding breast surgery and, as a result, be more proactive in deciding what's right for you. Finally, I hope that it helps you to get the most out of this new chapter in your life.

Cosmetic Breast
Surgery

Why Do You Want to Have Cosmetic Breast Surgery?

Right and Wrong Reasons for Going under the Knife

A FEW YEARS ago a woman named Meghan brought her husband into my office for her initial consultation for a breast enhancement or enlargement. The nurse had led them into the examination room and when I entered, my prospective patient was sitting in the examination chair and her husband was sitting on a swivel-back office chair in the corner. I introduced myself and began talking to her, as I always do, about her medical history and explained a bit about the procedures that I prefer for breast enlargements. When I reached the point in our discussion where I asked her what results she was hoping for from the surgery, her husband suddenly interrupted her.

"She wants them as big as you can make 'em—a double D," he piped in enthusiastically. Up until this point he had been sitting in the corner without making a sound.

I nodded slowly and looked at Meghan. She was just over

five feet tall and I doubt very much that she weighed over 105 pounds. "Well," I began, "I'm not going to try to discourage or encourage you from getting any particular cup size that you like, but I will ask you to consider the size relative to your body so that we can be sure of what really does look best for your body type."

"We're sure," said her husband, nodding vigorously. "Double D." Meghan looked down, perhaps a little bit embarrassed.

A doctor should not insert his own feelings into these matters, but it is important to be sure that a patient is fully aware of her options and that she is making her own decisions about her body only after careful consideration. I spoke directly to her, trying to elicit her opinions in the matter. "That's quite a large cup size for a woman of your proportions. Are you certain that you'd like to go that large?"

"I don't know. I guess . . ."

"She wants really big breasts," her husband broke in again. "What's so unusual about that? A lot of women want really big breasts."

"Okay," I said. "Fair enough. So you have a very clear idea about how you want your breasts to look . . ."

"Oh yeah!" said the husband.

"Yeah," she said with a worried look. In fact, she looked frightened. She looked scared to death.

"Can you make them so they stand really high? You know, like there's a bra, when there isn't a bra? And she wants them close together so that they have that natural cleavage . . ."

"Okay, okay," I said, raising a hand to quiet him before he got too carried away right there in my office. "I get it."

"Great!"

"But, unfortunately, I won't be able to help you."

The truth is that I knew within the first few minutes that I wasn't going to touch this young woman's body—and this is not an unusual story. There have been many times that I've decided not to operate on a patient that I felt had come to my office for all of the wrong reasons.

The following day, I spoke to Meghan on the telephone and told her that she was free to do as she liked, but that I hoped she'd spend time considering her own desires for her body. It seemed to me that she was having this procedure done for her husband and not at all for herself. I urged her to deeply consider not having this surgery for someone else, even if that someone else was her husband. On a purely emotional level, I really wanted to tell her to call a hotline for emotionally abused women or at least contact a psychologist. But I didn't. I told her that if some day she figured out what she wanted for herself, or if she had any other questions or concerns at all, that I'd be glad to speak with her again. I haven't heard from her and I can only assume that her husband found some other doctor who was willing to give him what he wanted.

SOCIAL PRESSURE

MUCH HAS BEEN made of the fact that of the body parts that we consider private—that we cover when we are in public—the breasts are the ones that are most noticeable. Much of a woman's experience through puberty is shaped by this obvious fact and while the formative years before the age of five may be the most important in determining how we will feel about ourselves in adulthood, our passage through puberty has got to run a close second. During puberty, no casual observer in the school hallway can tell if a boy's penis is developing yet or how large it is. (It's a good thing, too, because I don't think boys are emotionally strong enough to deal with that kind of thing). But for girls, their sexual development (or lack thereof) is obvious for everyone to see. Girls are teased if their breasts grow too early, too late, too big, too small. This kind of teasing during such a vulnerable period in life can create a desire to change to feel better about oneself.

Obviously no woman wants to be judged by her breast size, yet quite often women feel that breast size and proportions create an immediate, albeit unfair, impression. Frequently they are right. And there is a clear difference between judging a woman's breasts ("*Those are some beautiful breasts on that woman.*"), and judging a woman by her breasts ("*She's the woman with the beautiful breasts.*"). Even women who are exceptionally proud of their breasts should resent being defined in this second way.

The fact is that American society is obsessed with the female breast. Breasts are everywhere in popular culture, from advertisements to art, from adult entertainment to the stars that perform the music that our children listen to. And breasts have powerful symbolism for us, encompassing everything from sexual to nurturing aspects. The only place that you will find men famous for the size of their penis is in the world of pornography, whereas many women in popular culture are known for their breasts. This kind of pressure can make a woman feel self-conscious about herself, even when she has nothing to feel badly about. You can find more on this subject in Chapter Fourteen, "The Psychology of the Breast," by clinical psychologist, Dr. Jennifer N. Duffy.

DO IT FOR YOURSELF

BOTH MEN AND women want to be attractive to the opposite sex (or at least be attractive to whatever sex they are trying to attract). It has been my experience that, at least as far as men are concerned, there are as many who prefer women with small breasts as large. It would be a shame to either augment or reduce your breasts thinking that you will attract more men. You will only attract *different* men.

The only good reasons for having cosmetic breast surgery are *personal* reasons. It has to be about you—what *you* want and the *way* you want your body to be. Good reasons, bad reasons— only you can decide. I have often joked that my favorite patients are the ones whose husbands don't want them to do it. At least then I am confident that they are doing it for themselves.

Opting for cosmetic breast surgery is a very personal decision. Women arrive at the decision for many different reasons, but ultimately it should be a decision that you come to after deep thought and a real effort to gather the facts. I hope it's a deci- sion that you're really excited about and that afterwards it is a decision that you are truly pleased with. As with any important choice that you make about your future, there is no guarantee that you are not going to second-guess yourself years later, but there are a few factors that, if you think carefully about them now, will maximize your chances of being very happy later. Reading this book is your first step in that direction.

FACTORS TO CONSIDER

IF YOU ARE reading this book, then there is probably something that you don't like about your breasts. Here are some reasons that suggest that cosmetic breast surgery might be the right choice for you:

1. You think that your breasts are too small or too large. If this is the way you feel and you've felt this way for a long time and it really bothers you, then medical sci- ence can do something about it.
2. Your breasts have changed—because of weight loss, pregnancy, or just gravity—and you want your old breasts back again.
3. Your breasts are asymmetrical. It is completely normal

for one breast to be slightly different than the other, but sometimes the difference is so pronounced that it may make you very unhappy and shy.

4. You feel that your breasts are out of proportion with the rest of your body. It is amazing how different a woman's body can look by changing the size of her breasts to match her physique. For more on this, see the next chapter, "The Perfect Breasts."

5. You simply don't like the form of your breasts. Breasts not only vary in size, but in shape as well. Many women in great physical shape with otherwise attractive bodies have oddly shaped breasts. If this situation is embarrassing or otherwise burdensome for you, improvement can be made.

6. You have undergone a mastectomy or other injury to your breasts and want to repair or reconstruct them. One in eleven women have breast cancer at some time in their lives. Breast reconstruction after surgery is important to recovering not just from the illness, but also in recovering your life. I cover this in Chapter Thirteen, and there are several books devoted entirely to this subject.

7. You have had bad results from a previous surgery and want them fixed. I never like to belittle another surgeon's work or call them incompetent (though that certainly may be a factor in some cases), but even the best surgeons can sometimes end up with bad results. This is covered in Chapters Four ("Risks and Rewards") and Twelve ("Fixing Bad Surgery").

These are the most common reasons for contemplating cosmetic breast surgery, but certainly not the only ones.

There are also some factors that indicate that you should seriously reconsider having cosmetic breast surgery:

1. Your breasts are net yet fully developed. Cosmetic breast surgery is generally a big mistake for pubescent girls or any woman who is not fully developed. The exception would be a reduction for a girl who is suffering physical discomfort from her breast size. There is more on this subject in Chapter Nine, "Breast Reduction."

2. You are currently pregnant. You should not have the procedure if you are expecting. If you are planning to become pregnant in the very near future, it also makes sense to wait. Pregnancy and breast-feeding will probably change your breasts, even after surgery, and so it makes sense to get them done exactly as you would like afterwards.

3. If you are in a high-risk group for breast cancer. You should strongly consider not getting implant surgery. There is more specific information on this topic in Chapter Four, "Risks and Rewards."

4. You have unrealistic expectations of what can be achieved through this process. Improvement can almost always be achieved, but it isn't possible for every woman to have what she considers the "perfect breast." Reading this book is a good way to find out if your expectations are realistic.

There are many excellent arguments against having cosmetic surgery of any kind. Certainly there are always risks, and nobody should consider cosmetic surgery without carefully assessing the risks particular to the procedure they are contemplating. In the end, you must follow your own heart. No factor that helps you decide is wrong if it is your own.

Should We Remain the Way God Made Us?

I HAVE heard the argument that we should not try to improve upon God's design, but it could also be argued that it is God's intention that we strive to improve ourselves and the world in which we live. It is implicit in the adage that "God only helps those who help themselves." I have not noticed a great movement to reject vaccinations in order to die when God intends or to walk to work instead of drive in order to arrive when God intends. The use of scientific and technological progress to improve our lives is part of the human creative spirit that separates us from God's other creations.

The idea that cosmetic surgery is against God's design is not only hypocritical, but also frankly absurd. Does anyone believe that women with beautiful breasts were somehow chosen by God to be blessed in this way? Of course not! Furthermore, the same folks who argue against changing the appearance that you were born with are often wearing makeup and have styled their hair with electric blow dryers or curlers.

I have found tremendous satisfaction in my work helping women obtain the body that they truly want. You can do many things to change your body to your satisfaction—from dieting to working out. You can straighten or curl or change the color of your hair, you can even change the color of your eyes with contact lenses. But the only significant way to change the size and shape of your breasts is through cosmetic surgery. And the vast majority of women who have cosmetic breast surgery are afterwards not only very pleased with their breasts, but also with *themselves*. The most gratifying part of my job isn't improving a woman's body; it's improving her self-image.

Are there good reasons and bad reasons to embark on this journey? Well, that's a necessarily subjective matter. As I've stated, if the reasons are personal, that is, the reasons make sense to you, then it would be impossible for anyone to argue that they are *bad* reasons. After years as a plastic surgeon with countless patients, and knowing so many women who are pleased with their decisions and a few who are not, I believe that the *best* reason to embark on this journey is to feel better about yourself. It is those women who, after careful consideration of all of the factors, risks, and rewards, believe that they will both be happier with themselves and will have a better self-image after the surgery that will ultimately get the most out of this process and are most likely to be pleased with the results.

The Perfect Breasts

Brazil versus Texas

IS THERE SUCH a thing as the perfect breast? I won't keep you in suspense. The answer is no.

The idea of the perfect breast has changed, sometimes with blinding rapidity, many times throughout history—from place to place, culture to culture, and individual to individual.

Nothing illustrates this better than a patient named Donna. When I first met Donna she lived in Texas with her second husband and two children and worked as a paralegal in a prestigious law firm in Dallas. Years earlier, as a fairly famous beauty queen, she had won numerous pageants and awards, and she was still an exceptionally beautiful woman. But after two children, her breasts had never returned to their former shape, and she had heard my name through a friend and decided to fly out to New York to have her breasts done at my office in Manhattan. Once you are having surgery, you may as well get exactly what you want, so Donna opted to have implants that were substantially larger than her breasts had been prior to her pregnancies. I'm pleased to report that she was delighted with the results and told me that she felt better about herself and received more compliments about her body than she had even when she had been competing in beauty pageants.

A few years later, Donna moved to New York City. Her husband was offered a great job there and Donna found a corporate law firm that was willing to hire her for far more than she was being paid in Dallas. Everything was so exciting for them as they started new lives in Manhattan. And then a strange thing happened. After being on the social "A-list" for years in Dallas, Donna began to feel out of place in the more conservative world of New York lawyers and high society. It was a new place and culture with very different fashions and ideals of beauty than Donna was used to. Instead of making her feel confident and beautiful, her very large breasts made her feel self-conscious, unsophisticated, and awkward.

And so Donna once again returned to my office—this time to have her implants replaced with much *smaller* ones, along with a small lift, giving her a smaller cup size than her natural breasts had been. This story has a happy ending: Donna still lives in New York with her family and loves her job, her life, and her body.

Also, Donna's story has a moral, one that is applicable to anyone: You tend to buy into the ideals of the people around you. It has nothing to do with being weak willed or easily influenced by others. Think about the way your own tastes have changed over the years and then take a look at what you see on television, the movies, and in the advertisements all around you. We all respond to some extent to the aesthetic norms around us. I call this the Brazil versus Texas Effect, because nowhere are the two extremes of desired breast types more evident.

Both Brazil and Texas are places where there are a very high number of women seeking cosmetic breast surgery. But the surgery they are seeking is the opposite. In Texas, many women are looking for **augmentation**, and most of those women are opting for rather large implants. In Brazil, almost all of the women are having reductions or lifts. On the topless beaches of Rio, the girl who turns the most heads is the one with pert, usually tiny breasts.

So what are the perfect breasts for you? Overwhelmingly the answer to that question is: the perfect breasts for you are whatever you want them to be! But wait, before you point to a picture in a magazine and say, "those are the breasts for me," consider this: Every woman in the world has a girlfriend whose favorite color is, let's say green, who looks terrible whenever she wears green. In other words, although those large implants may look great on someone else, it doesn't mean that you will be as lucky! So there are some other factors you might want to consider before deciding what you want your breasts to look like.

CONSIDERING THE PERFECT BREASTS

IT MAY SOUND obvious, but symmetry is a key consideration in choosing what you want your breasts to look like, and by what procedure you intend to achieve that look. In my experience you will be happier with a procedure that addresses symmetry before size concerns. Sometimes correcting **asymmetry** is easily achieved by using two different sized implants (in the case of an augmentation) or removing different amounts of tissue from each breast (as in the case of a lift or reduction). In many cases, enlarging the breasts may increase the appearance of a small lack of symmetry. For example, if one breast points slightly further toward the outside and the other more forward, implants will increase that disparity, making the breasts appear very mismatched. If a woman is still very intent on dramatically increasing the size of her breast, other sculpting surgery might be recommended, such as relocating the **nipple-areola complex** or some sculpting **liposuction**.

Another major consideration is proportion. Breasts that you admire on another woman might look wrong on you. If you want to maintain a very natural look, this should be a consideration. Proportion is also important in balancing the overall look you want to achieve for your entire body. For example, a woman with large hips who wants a dramatic reduction in breast size might be surprised by how much larger her hips appear after surgery. Likewise, a woman with narrow hips might be advised to consider what her bottom will look like after large implants. In figure 1 the hips are exactly the same size in both women. Without the added chest width of augmentation, the hips on the left appear larger and out of proportion. Conversely, a woman with wide hips can expect an improvement in body proportions by adding upper body width.

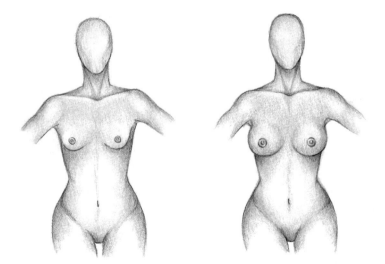

These two models of equal hip width demonstrate the overall balance of upper torso and lower body. Note the imbalance of the upper body in the model with small breasts (on the left). Despite the equal dimensions of the hip width, the patient with the smaller breasts appears to have larger hips.

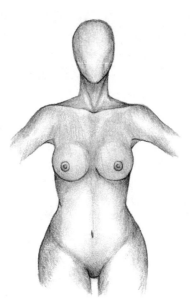

In an effort to accentuate cleavage, many implants are placed too close together on the chest wall. Note the imbalance of the upper body with large medial cleavage and absence of lateral chest break. Also, the implants necessary to create this look will most likely cause the nipples to point outward.

There is also the question of **lateral chest break**, or the appearance of the breasts protruding past the rib cage on each side as seen in silhouette from the front. Often women request implants that are placed in such a way that their breasts will be close together so that they will have "natural" cleavage. In fact, nothing could be less natural. Natural looking breasts fall slightly to the sides. Cleavage is the result of natural looking breasts that are pressed together in a bra or bodice. Each woman is entitled to make her own decision about what she wants, but if she wants her breasts to look natural, she should consider this. Also, breasts that have a lateral break will attractively enhance proportion as discussed above. If the breasts are close together and protrude straight out in front, it will cause the hips to appear unnaturally wide. In the illustrations below, the woman's hips and breasts are the same size, but in the first illustration the breasts are unnaturally close together and in the second she has a natural looking lateral chest break, making the rest of her body appear to be more in proportion.

What about the shape of the breasts? For most people who have never considered cosmetic breast surgery, beautiful breasts are simply "breast shaped." In fact beautiful breasts come in many different shapes, and different individuals are likely to be attracted to different shapes. Beyond the consideration of size, some breasts are much rounder and some more oval shaped. Generally, rounder breasts are considered less "natural" looking, but some women are born that way. Again, different types of implants and different procedures yield a different shape of breast, so it's important to know what shape you are looking for.

Now let's talk about nipples. A large part of the overall look of your breasts is determined by the position, size (diameter of the **areola**), and how much they stick out (nipple projection). As always, these are all a matter of personal preference. For a very natural looking breast, the nipple should be positioned slightly to the outside of the breast at the point where the breast rises farthest from the body (the point of greatest projection). Some women will prefer them slightly higher on the breast, yet this position often gives a "bottomed-out" look with more breast volume below the nipple. The nipple tends to point upward instead of forward.

When considering areola diameter, studies suggest that the ideal areola is between forty-two and forty-five millimeters across. Some women prefer larger, some smaller, but there are other considerations that have to do with the procedure that you choose. For example, it may be impossible to give you a very small areola diameter in order to avoid a secondary scar

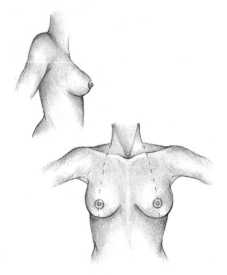

The perfect breasts are a misnomer. Aesthetic and pleasing breasts, regardless of size, are well balanced. This illustration refers to a nipple-areola complex on the midpoint of the breast mound, slightly outside a line drawn from the outside border of the neck to the floor. Breast volume should be equal on the inside and outside of the nipple.

below the nipple in the case of lift. In the case of an augmentation, as the skin of the breast is stretched to accommodate the implant, the width of the areola is likely to increase proportionally and you may (or may not) want it trimmed down at the same time. There is more detail on both of these considerations in the chapters on breast reduction and breast augmentation, respectively.

Other considerations in achieving the "perfect breast" might include addressing excess skin or sagging breast tissue. Extra skin and sagging breast tissue are directly related to breast **ptosis**. Ptosis (pronounced *toe-sis*) refers to the weakening of the ligaments that hold the breasts up—basically, breast ptosis just means sagging breasts. For some women this is the result of aging, breast-feeding, large weight loss, or gravity, but for many young women sagging is also commonplace from the onset of puberty—they are simply the breasts that they were born with!

Excess fat may affect the shape of the breast or create the folds that appear under the arms alongside the breasts when wearing a bra or the folds that appear above the bra, just above the armpits. One of my patients, referring to this axillary fat, coined the term "chicken nuggets." These are usually eliminated with liposuction and this technique can drastically improve the final look of your breasts.

What Are Perfect Breasts?

BECAUSE the perfect breasts are a matter of opinion, I have seen many women in my office that I didn't think needed any work on their breasts at all. Many women who are considering cosmetic breast surgery are going to hear that opinion. Some of the people that tell you that your breasts are perfect just the way they are may be coming from a place of politics or social values, but some of them might honestly like the way they look as they are. Some women may even think that your breasts are the perfect breasts that they wish that they were born with. Nobody can tell a woman that she does or does not need to change her appearance—to do so is either arrogant, condescending, or both. The decision is not grounded in facts, but rather in emotion.

IT'S UP TO YOU

THE CONSIDERATIONS I have just discussed mainly deal with finding the right breasts for your body. But still, it is and must be an emotional decision. So, to return to the example of your friend whose favorite color is green, she may discover that she looks best when she wears yellows and golds. But if she really loves green, that may outweigh other considerations and she may decide she's going to wear green anyway. Likewise, it is perfectly reasonable for a woman to decide that she wants a particular size or shape of breast regardless of whether or not it looks natural on her body. By now I may be sounding like a broken record, but it bears repeating: Only you can decide what you want your body to look like. The only aesthetic limitations should come not from the tastes of your friends or family or even your doctor, but from the limitations of medical science.

Once you have decided exactly how you would like your breasts to look, it is time make a game plan. There may be several different surgical techniques available to achieve the desired results, so many decisions are still ahead. Some procedures have a much better chance of giving you the shape you want but may involve more risk, increased scarring, or other undesirable results. Other procedures will not be as satisfying, but will be safe and reliable. The difficulty of your decision will depend both on what your breasts look like now and what you want your breasts to look like afterwards.

In the following chapters, I will take you step-by-step through the different procedures and tell you what you can expect, as well as the unique risks related to each. First, let's begin by looking at all of your major options.

What Are Your Options?

The Nonsurgical and Surgical Basics

IN THIS CHAPTER, I will begin by discussing all of the non-surgical options available as alternatives to cosmetic breast surgery. Many of these options have some merit, but others are snake oil. This chapter is a must read for anyone tempted to order miracle breast enlargement cream from the back cover of her favorite tabloid. I'll begin this discussion with women who are interested in having their breasts smaller, lifted, or re-shaped, because for these women there are few options other than surgery.

NON-SURGICAL OPTIONS FOR BREAST REDUCTION

IF YOU ARE considering breast reduction, the first option that you should consider is weight loss—assuming, of course, that you are currently overweight. There are many thin women with very large breasts that are out of proportion to their bodies. Trying to starve yourself to reduce your cup size under those circumstances could be dangerous, and at minimum, you'd want to consult your doctor before embarking on such a regimen. However, if you are currently overweight, it makes sense to try to lose the weight naturally before considering breast reduction surgery. It is unlikely that you will achieve the results that you desire because much of the breast tissue might not be fat at all. But you can always opt for surgery later if your breasts do not reduce to your satisfaction. Furthermore, there are many health risks associated with being overweight that are far more important than breast size. People who are overweight do not live as long and are more susceptible to a large range of diseases—including, by the way, breast cancer—than people who live within a healthy weight range.

There are, obviously, limits to how much weight loss will affect breast size. It may have no affect at all! And if you are a woman who suffers from a multitude of physical symptoms (back pain, shoulder notching, neck pain, or rashes under your breasts) because your breasts are simply too large, your best option may very well be surgical breast reduction. Furthermore, if you are also concerned about ptosis, or the sagging of your breasts, there is nothing that weight loss can do about that. In fact, weight loss might make the sagging worse. (*Please* don't misconstrue this to mean that you shouldn't lose weight if you are overweight.) The myriad benefits to your body and health from weight loss far exceed in importance any changes in the appearance of your breasts!

There are all sorts of exercise programs out there that falsely tout their ability to lift or reduce your breast size. I am sorry to inform you that they are all false claims. There is no exercise that can lift your breasts, and exercise can only reduce the size of your breasts in as far as it aids you in losing weight.

Unfortunately, as you lose weight, your breasts may begin to sag even further. However, like weight loss, there are many important benefits to exercise that have nothing to do with your breasts. Everyone should exercise. According to one of the latest studies, a lack of exercise is a more dangerous factor in determining how long and how well you live than either obesity or even *smoking*! So again, I would stress that the benefits of regular exercise are more important than the look of your breasts. Though exercise cannot significantly change the appearance of your breasts, it turns out that there may still be some relationship between the two. To find out more about that relationship read the next chapter on risks and rewards.

NONSURGICAL OPTIONS FOR BREAST ENLARGEMENT

FOR BREAST ENLARGEMENT, there are a few more options and I will take a moment now to examine some of the products that you may have seen on the market.

▷ Pills and Creams

On late night infomercials and everywhere on the Internet there are many companies that sell various pills and creams to increase the size of your breasts. Some of them even promise an increase of two-cup sizes! They are as real as the X-ray glasses sold in the back of comic books. While these very slick companies talk a very good game, there is currently no evidence that they do anything whatsoever. Most offer money-back guarantees and have all sorts of testimonials from women who have had the greatest success with these products that make them seem very credible, but in fact they are merely taking advantage of sneaky, well-known marketing ploys.

Beware of Internet Scams!

DISREPUTABLE as well as reputable companies selling breast-enlargement products will often offer money-back guarantees because of well-known marketing studies that indicate that customers—even those who say that the guarantee was one of the main reasons for their purchase—will very rarely attempt to get their money back *even if they are dissatisfied with the product*. Because it's just too much of a hassle, they usually let it go. For the few clients who actually pursue getting their money back, the companies consider that a small cost of doing business.

As for testimonials from women who claim that the product has worked for them, small disclaimers like "results not typical," or "you may not do as well," allow these companies to legally make even the most outrageous claims. These disclaimers are not intended to protect you, the consumer, but to protect them, the companies, from lawsuits.

Infomercials are not policed in the same way as regular television sponsorship commercials. Whereas any false claim on a regular television commercial can lead to swift penalties from the Federal Trade Commission (FTC), infomercials have established their own, self-governing body, called the National Infomercial Marketing Association (NIMA), to eliminate false claims. In order to qualify for certification under NIMA, infomercials must not make any false claims. But there is currently no requirement to actually obtain this certification. Disreputable companies merely run their infomercials without obtaining certification from NIMA.

As for the Internet—well, as everyone knows, the Internet is cowboy country. There is so much false and even illegal material on the Internet that it is impossible for any government agency to maintain any degree of control. The FBI does not even seem able to control the propagation of child pornography. How can they possibly deal with the myriad of illegitimate business practices? Hundreds of websites quote studies and make unbelievable claims, all of which are completely fictional, and law enforcement is either unwilling or unable to keep up with them. Whenever doing business with an Internet company, you should check their rating on Gomez.com (a company that rates the reliability of websites) or look for a website that has the approval of the Better Business Bureau, signified by the BBBOnline seal. With this said, there are many reputable websites sponsored by non-profit organizations that will honestly help you in your search for information. See the Internet resource section in the back of the book for some reliable websites that you may find helpful.

The simple fact is that if pills or creams actually worked they would have to be regulated by the FDA. However, if for some reason you should still want to experiment with these pills and creams, I would recommend the creams, as you are less likely to have some sort of dangerous allergic reaction to the ingredients, and since they must be rubbed onto the breast, you might at least have some fun using them!

There is one pill that is regulated by the FDA that might give you some small increase in breast size: birth control pills. Most women who begin a regimen of birth control pills report a small increase in overall body weight (usually five to ten pounds) that is accompanied by a small increase in breast size (usually not significant enough to create a need for a new bra size).

▷ The Brava

There is only one other device that I know of that is publicly marketed to women to increase their breast size. The **Brava** uses a sophisticated suction device that is applied to your chest over a ten-week period to permanently enlarge the breasts. The good news is that it works without the need for any surgery or scars. The bad news is two-fold: There are currently no long-term studies as to any dangerous side effects of this process, and the results are very limited.

The device itself consists of two plastic domes that are worn over the breasts and a small electronic pump that maintains a slight suction inside the domes. The domes are worn for ten hours every day for ten weeks. Because of the somewhat bulky nature of the apparatus, most women choose to wear it at night, beginning a few hours before bed and then removing it in the morning.

As of January, 2004, women who wish to try the Brava suction device must do so as part of a study group. To become eligible for the study group, you must first submit a questionnaire and health history to the company, which may be completed through its website. Though it is a study, the participating women are required to pay for the apparatus and the continuing health care which is monitored by the company and its physicians—and it is quite expensive.

Why the study? It may be that the device is perfectly safe, but there are many credible voices in the scientific community, myself included, who are alarmed by the prospect that it may increase the risk of breast cancer. Again, to be fair, I'd like to stress that no studies have yet been completed so there is no current indication that the device might increase cancer risk. The risk is only theoretical and is based on the idea of "loss of **contact inhibition**."

Contact inhibition is the mechanism inside cells that tells them when to stop multiplying. Scientists aren't sure exactly how this mechanism works, but it is considered one of the keys to figuring out the mysteries of cancer. Normal cells will stop multiplying when in direct contact with other cells of their kind.

Cancer is formed when cells don't behave in this normal manner and continue to multiply out of control. The fear with the suction device is that in order to make the breasts grow, it causes the cells of the breast tissue to lose their contact inhibition. In other words, the cells temporarily behave in a manner similar to cancer cells. Could this be a risk factor in an area of the body that is frequently prone to problems with cancerous growth? Nobody yet has the long-term answers to that question. In the short term, it seems to pose no risk, but the same can be said of sunburn, which can sometimes initiate a cancerous growth twenty years later.

The other problem with the suction device is that you do not get much in return for your risk. You do get natural breast growth of natural breast tissue, but the most growth that can be achieved with the Brava device is about 100 or maybe 120 cubic centimeters (ccs). When you consider that the smallest implants used for even the most petite women seeking the most subtle enlargement in breast size is about 200 ccs, you can see that this does not represent a very significant enlargement for most women.

Is this suction device right for you? Only you can decide. If you have no family history of breast cancer and you are willing to take an unknown risk to avoid going under the knife and if you have only the most minimal expectations for enlargement, it may be worth a try.

▷ Exercise

There are also exercise regimens that you may encounter to expand your breasts. Again, I will stress the benefits of exercise, but even with a substantial amount of work to expand your **pectoral muscles** (the muscles beneath the breasts) you will not see any significant results to the breast itself. Women who are serious body-builders will see the pectoral muscle bulging above their breasts, just beneath the collarbone.

CHOOSING SURGERY

ONCE YOU HAVE considered the choices that I have just discussed, there are two remaining options. One is to be satisfied with your body and do nothing, and the other is to opt for cosmetic breast surgery.

If you choose cosmetic breast surgery, another universe of viable options opens up for you. The rest of this book deals with the many options that you will face in this process and will serve as a guide in helping you make the most informed decisions. Actually, the best way to begin is to backwards. First, decide what you want your end result to be and then figure out which procedure(s) will give you the result you are looking for.

In brief, your surgical options can be generalized to include lifts, reductions, implants, and "sculpting" techniques. To achieve the result that you desire may require a combination of all of these techniques. For example, some women after breast-feeding are left with sagging, very flattened breasts. A woman in this situation might want to consider both a breast lift and an implant to restore the shape of her breasts. I have devoted a separate chapter to each of these general options for cosmetic breast surgery. But before you make your decision about which procedures are right for you there is one more thing that every patient must consider: What are the risk factors associated with cosmetic breast surgery?

Risks and Rewards

Don't Pass "Go" Until You Read This!

THIS MAY BE the most important chapter in this book, and I hope that you read it carefully. If you could improve the appearance of your breasts without any risk or cost, it would be a very simple decision indeed! You could make them larger for that revealing evening gown and then reduce them for exercise class the next morning. If it could only be so. In the real world, breast surgery comes at certain costs and uncertain risks.

Each procedure has its own individual inherent risks, and I will try to address all of them, but it must be understood that there may be other risks that are not covered here or that science simply does not yet know about.

COSTS

LET'S BEGIN WITH the basics: the definite financial costs that come with surgery. As of January 2004, there are almost no cosmetic procedures that are covered under medical insurance. The exceptions are reconstruction after **mastectomy** and some reductions in women who suffer secondary complications of their breast size such as severe back and neck pain or traumatic skin problems from chaffing. So, unless you fall into one of those categories, you should be prepared to spend quite a bit of money for the surgery. If you are currently uninsured, you should also be prepared for the possibility of additional costs for any treatment necessary in the event of complications resulting from the surgery. Furthermore, if you do experience complications from your surgery, it is possible that this will make it more difficult or more expensive to obtain medical insurance coverage in the future.

Although insurance will not cover your cosmetic procedure, the company is prohibited by law to drop your policy in the event of complications. However, to be as prudent as possible, I advise you to find out from your current provider exactly what the rules are regarding cosmetic breast surgery before you proceed.

While the monetary price of your procedure is perhaps the most obvious and definite cost to cosmetic breast surgery, it should be obvious that bargain hunting is not a good idea where any surgery is concerned. The next chapter deals with finding a surgeon, and though cost may ultimately be a realistic factor in your choice, it is not a factor that is discussed in that chapter. There are too many other factors that are so much more important for you and your health. In fact, the main factor in minimizing all of the other risk factors is finding the right surgeon.

The Price of a New Chest

ALTHOUGH prices will vary based on the region of the country as well as the experience of your surgeon, here are rough estimates for the costs of the different procedures:

Breast Reduction	$6,000-12,000
Breast Augmentation	$4,000-8,000
Breast Lift	$5,000-10,000

PAIN

ANOTHER FACTOR THAT you should think of as a given is that you will suffer a certain amount of pain during recovery. How much pain you experience will depend both upon you and your body and also upon what kind of procedure you opt for. You may be able to get a more definitive idea of what you are in for by speaking candidly with your surgeon; however, each woman is unique and it is impossible to know how much pain you will experience. In addition, I don't find it helpful to talk about the pain with friends who have had cosmetic breast surgery, as quite often two similar patients will describe significant differences in the amount of pain they encounter.

Don't Say I Didn't Warn You!

IT IS important to make preparations in the event that your procedure turns out more painful than usual. As an extreme example, one of my patients who opted for a **submuscular** breast augmentation (a procedure that yields beautiful results, but is frequently quite painful during recovery), related the following story:

When she left the recovery room with her boyfriend she was feeling fine, but in the cab on the way home, the bumping and shifting of the taxi on New York's famously potholed and rutted streets became so painful that she could not continue the ride. She told the driver to stop and pull over. It would be better to walk than to bear this agony for another moment. She and her boyfriend got out of the cab. They were only two blocks from home, but after a few steps, she quickly realized that walking was going to be impossible, too. She sat down on the curb and began to cry while her boyfriend tried to figure out what to do. The young man was at his wits' end with worry when he suddenly had an idea. He made a quick call on his cell phone and found a limousine company that could send a car immediately. Within minutes, a big, stretch Cadillac arrived and he gently helped her into the back of the vehicle. They gave the driver special instructions to go very slowly, at little more than a crawl, and they made it home. It was probably the most expensive two-block ride that anyone has ever taken.

Of course when my patient told me this story I felt terrible. She looked puzzled by this and said, "Doc, you told me in advance that it was going to hurt and I appreciated your honesty. I should have prepared better to deal with it." She went on to say that she still considered the surgery the best decision of her life and she would do it again in a moment, but the next time she would be sure to listen to all of the doctor's recommendations regarding the possibility of a painful recovery.

Along with pain you can also expect some swelling and black-and-blue, as well as general unpleasantness (dried blood around the dressings and uncomfortable bras). Again, this depends a great deal on the procedure and on the individual. Certainly some women experience these problems much less than others. But you should expect that for at least the first few days, you breasts will not look very appealing at all. This is no indication of how they will ultimately appear, but even when the final result is perfect, this period of healing is something that you must be prepared for nonetheless. Planning a vacation to the beach for the week after your surgery would obviously be unwise.

IT'S PERMANENT

ANOTHER FACTOR THAT you must consider carefully is that cosmetic breast surgery is fundamentally irreversible. If you change your mind afterwards you can never return your body to the way it was before surgery. It is possible to have subsequent surgeries to improve or to simply re-alter the appearance of your breasts, and it *may* even be possible to return them substantially to the way they looked before the surgery, but you must go into this decision with the mindset that this is a one-way ticket. For example, if you have a substantial enlargement and later choose to have the implants removed, the stretched skin and tissue that is left behind will result in sagging of the breast. While this might be corrected by a surgical re-sculpting and/or breast lift, it may result in additional scarring and increase the risks of additional complications. No woman should ever opt to have breast surgery merely to see what it will look like. Before you make your final decision you must be certain that this is something you want for your body, and you must be prepared to live with the results.

SCARRING

THE LAST OF the definite risk factors associated with cosmetic breast surgery is scarring. While different procedures will result in different types, shapes, and placement of scars, and while some scars can be very well hidden, there is no way to have surgery without any scars at all. Once you and your surgeon have decided exactly what procedure will yield the closest results to what you want, you will have to decide if living with the scars is acceptable to you. For more on exactly what kind and how much scarring you might end up with, you can read the subsequent chapters on each type of procedure.

Keep in mind that different individuals have different scarring and healing potential. Often very light or very dark skinned women will scar more visibly. By observing scars of old injuries from your childhood you may get some indication of your body's resistance to visible scarring. Post-operative treatments designed to minimize the scarring and redness are advisable and discussed in Chapter Twelve, "Fixing Bad Surgery."

DISSATISFACTION AND COMPLICATIONS

THE FACTORS I'VE just described represent the problems that you will encounter with any cosmetic breast procedure, even with the best possible outcome. But there are many other problems that might also arise if things don't go perfectly. The most obvious of these is cosmetic dissatisfaction—not liking the way your breasts came out.

There are many ways that you can be dissatisfied with the appearance of your breasts after surgery. For example, you may not be happy about the size, the shape, the location of the nipples, or the symmetry of your breasts. In addition there's possible scarring or, in the case of implants, **capsular contracture** (see page 39), rippling, or the outline of the implant being visible beneath the skin. The best way to avoid being unhappy about the results of your surgery is to make sure that you and your surgeon are communicating effectively. If you feel unsure that your doctor understands what you are saying, don't just hope for the best. It would be a mistake to think that just because your doctor has done this procedure thousands of times that she or he probably knows how you would like to look. A plastic surgeon has many techniques that result in a wide variety of outcomes. It is up to you to inform your doctor to the best of your ability *exactly* what you are hoping for. Don't put yourself in the position of making yourself clear *after* the surgery.

Also ensure that your surgeon is communicating effectively with you. Make sure that you understand what you are being told. Remember that there are realistic limits to the process, so you must be realistic in your expectations. Not every woman is a good candidate for every procedure. Just because surgeons can make some other woman's breasts look a certain way doesn't mean that they can do the same for you, especially if they are starting with a very different breast or body type to begin with. If three surgeons tell you that it is unlikely that they can achieve a certain look for you without unacceptable scarring and a fourth says, "Well, why don't we try it and see?" you should take this as a very bad signal. Don't become somebody's guinea pig. Remember: Even the simplest procedures can, in rare cases, go wrong.

Even though a bad result is unlikely, it is important to know exactly what could go wrong. Some of the complications that might occur include the development of a **hematoma**, infection, **seroma**, tissue **necrosis**, and complications arising from **anesthesia**.

A hematoma is nothing more than a collection of blood inside the body. A bruise is a simple hematoma beneath the skin. In most cases a small hematoma will simply reabsorb itself into the body, but if the hematoma is larger or is not being reabsorbed properly, your surgeon will probably choose to **aspirate** it—which means that he or she will insert a small needle and drain away the collection of blood. This should be a very simple procedure that will not cause any additional scarring. More significant hematomas may require surgical intervention to remove all of the hematoma and possibly stop any active bleeding that is causing the blood to accumulate. Under normal circumstances, moderate hematomas are not a big deal other than the inconvenience of an additional office visit, but again, it is important that you communicate well with your doctor about any unusual pain, tenderness, or swelling so that it can be dealt with properly. A large hematoma left untreated could cause other problems, such as infection and/or increased capsular contracture, resulting in distortion of the shape and hardening of the implant.

Any time you open up the skin you are at risk for an infection. Modern surgical and sterilization techniques are truly excellent, so the chances of infection are now extremely low. But the possibility always exists that some kind of microbe will sneak in either during the procedure or later during the early stages of recovery. It is important that you follow all of your surgeon's recommendations regarding the treatment of the incision sites to maintain a clean and protected environment for your healing to take place. Most infections that are a result of surgery will show symptoms within a few days of the surgery. Signs of infection include redness or a sunburn-like rash, swelling, pain, or unusual discharge, and, most obviously, a fever. If you have any suspicion of an infection, and especially if you encounter a fever a few days after surgery, it is important to see your doctor.

An infection, like a hematoma, is usually no big deal as long as it is dealt with in a timely manner. Usually a simple round of antibiotics will fix the problem. However, infections associated with an implant may be harder to treat than those with normal body tissue, and if the antibiotics fail to resolve the problem the implant may have to be removed. A new implant can be placed after the infection is completely gone. In very rare circumstances, **toxic shock syndrome (TSS)** is also a possibility. Symptoms of TSS include rash, fever, diarrhea, vomiting, fainting, and dizziness. TSS is a potentially lethal condition so if you have any suspicion that you display the symptoms described above, *immediately* see your surgeon.

Swelling is a well-known component of all surgeries, as well as most lumps and bumps. Swelling is the result of local tissue fluid, known as **serum**, leaving the bloodstream and entering into the space around cells. After surgery, serum may fill the space created by the incisions and reduced or sculpted breast tissue. In most cases this fluid is self-limited or is removed by drains, but in some cases it creates a persistent swelling known as a seroma, which requires frequent aspirations until accumulation ceases. This is usually more of a nuisance than a problem. However, in rare instances this problem can lead to infection.

Left untreated, complications like a hematoma, seroma, or an infection can result in more serious complications that may require hospitalization, or even tissue necrosis. This is bad stuff. The word *necrosis* is Greek and actually means "death," and tissue necrosis literally means that a portion of the skin breast tissue, or other affected area has died. This is usually the result of a severe infection or a decrease of blood supply to the area. Cigarette smoking is a risk factor that makes the chance of tissue necrosis rise significantly by reducing blood supply to all tissues. So, a word of warning: Don't Smoke! If you sustain tissue necrosis after surgery, it may require the excision (removal) of the affected tissue. Necrosis is very rare, but it may be more common in cases where there has been previous or bad surgery or in cases of breast reconstruction where the blood supply to the tissue has already been compromised. It is critical that your surgeon takes into account any previous surgery on your breasts in these circumstances so that all care can be taken to protect the remaining blood supply. If a large area of breast tissue or part of the nipple develops necrosis after the tissue is removed, it may require further surgical reconstruction that may result in further scarring.

ANESTHESIA'S RISKS

ANOTHER COMMON RISK to all surgery is related to the greatest miracle of modern surgery: anesthesia. There was a time not so very long ago when surgeons had to operate with nothing more than a shot of whiskey to ease the pain of patients. Even surgery that we consider simple and routine today often resulted in death from shock. With the use of local and general anesthesia, a new world emerged for surgeons.

Today, the techniques of the modern anesthesiologist are unsurpassed and anesthesia is far safer than even just a few years ago. There are long and careful protocols to ensure your safety and your vital signs will be carefully monitored not only before and during your surgery but afterwards as well to ensure that everything is working perfectly as you emerge from the effects of the anesthesia. With today's technology, the anesthesia may well be a less dangerous portion of your surgery than the drive to your doctor's office.

If you plan on checking out your surgeon, you might want to find out about your surgeon's anesthesiologist as well. Many surgeons opt for a nurse anesthetist as a way of cutting costs. Many nurse anesthetists are extremely competent, and they have extensive and excellent training, however, I personally only perform surgery with a board certified anesthesiologist. I believe that even if the difference is minor, it is worth minimizing every possible risk to your health and safety. It is important to emphasize that if you have *ever* had *any* complications with, or unexpected reactions to anesthesia in the past or you have reason to believe you might in the future, you must communicate this to your surgeon.

Another component of the overall risk profile of the procedure will be the operative facility. Is it an accredited facility? Is it certified to perform the type of surgery and anesthesia you are having? If you are electing to have the procedure in a hospital these questions are moot, because all hospitals are required to undergo strict examinations. In-office procedures, however are another issue entirely. While many office operating rooms are accredited by one of several governing boards, many are not. It is important to question your physician as to the type and degree of accreditation of any office-based facility. If the facility you will have your surgery in is accredited by the **AAAASF**, **AAHC**, **JACHO**, or Medicare, the facility has passed stringent guidelines and its safety has been demonstrated.

SPECIFIC RISKS ASSOCIATED WITH IMPLANTS

THE RISK FACTORS that I have discussed thus far are the general risk factors associated with cosmetic breast surgery. Now I will discuss risks specifically associated with breast implants. These risks are *in addition* to the other risks stated above.

Breast implants are made from a **silicone** polymer bag that has been filled with either saline (saltwater) or **silicone gel,** and they are used in breast augmentation or enlargement procedures to increase breast size. There are several risk factors associated directly with implants that you should be aware of before considering breast augmentation.

I have already mentioned the first risk factor: cosmetic dissatisfaction. There are a few things specific to implants that might lead you to become disappointed in the way your breasts look after surgery. The most obvious has to do with size. It is very important to think long and hard not just about how large you want your breasts to be, but how those breasts will look on your body. I will discuss this further in Chapter Seven, "Breast

Enlargement," but for now I will say that many women think in terms of cup size or implant volume when they should be thinking about *proportion*.

Another cosmetic risk that is possible with implants is seeing the edge of the implant through the skin. This is most common with the **subglandular** procedure (which is also discussed further Chapter Seven), however, it is always a possibility and may occur even in great looking augmented breasts when viewed in certain positions or from certain angles. Additionally, in some cases, particularly with the use of *textured* implants, a ripple on the surface of the breast may appear when you turn your body or lie on your side.

Asymmetry is another possible cause of cosmetic dissatisfaction. This might result from certain procedures that make it difficult to place the implants in exactly the same position on both sides or as a result of the implants shifting after surgery. Overzealous surgical dissection can cause the implant to move down or down and out (toward the armpit). Asymmetry is also a common result of rotation or displacement of **anatomical** (teardrop-shaped) **implants**. When round implants rotate nothing happens to the result because a rotated circle is still a circle. The teardrop-shape implants however, have a discrete shape with an asymmetrical axis. If an anatomical implant rotates on one side but not the other, the asymmetry will be obvious and very disconcerting.

A cause of major cosmetic dissatisfaction with implants is a problem known as **pectoral shelf deformity**. Many women that I have seen in my practice who asked me to fix a previous surgery came because of pectoral shelf deformity. This problem occurs when the implant protrudes from the top of the breast tissue so that the breast seems to fall beneath the implant and the top of the implant is clearly visible beneath the skin.

CAPSULAR CONTRACTURE

THE LAST CAUSE of possible cosmetic dissatisfaction and perhaps the most important is a risk factor with implants that can be its own little universe of troubles: capsular contracture. Capsular contracture is a common problem with implants and probably the one that you've heard about, maybe even heard some horror stories about, so I'm going to spend some time now discussing what it is, what it can mean for you, and what the odds are of it happening to you if you have a breast augmentation.

It may surprise you to learn that your chances of getting some amount of capsular formation are 100 percent. The formation of a capsule around the implant is simply a normal and unavoidable response from your body. The capsule itself is like a form of scar tissue and can be rigid. In most cases the formation of this capsule is harmless and in some ways beneficial in that it holds the implant in place. The problems arise when the capsule grows too thick and begins to contract tightly around the implant. Since all women with breast implants will experience varying degrees of capsular contracture, a scale was developed to describe the amount of capsule formation present and how adversely it affects the patient. This scale, known as the **Baker Scale**, has four levels or classes:

- ○ **Baker Class I** refers to the minimum level of capsular contracture. Breasts are considered Class I if the capsule formation is so minor that it can neither be seen nor felt at all. This is the best possible outcome.
- ○ **Baker Class II** means that even though you can't see any difference in the breast, you will be able to feel the capsule as a hardening of the implant. This may be a very subtle change or a very obvious hardening. I often

describe this as a feeling of wax paper wrapped around the implant.

- ○ **Baker Class III** is when you can both feel and see the difference in the implant because of the capsule formation. The capsule might be quite firm and the appearance may manifest as a ripple in the surface or a change in the shape of the implant as the capsule contracts around it. This change in shape may make the implant look smaller or it may appear to move higher on the chest. In my experience, most implants do not actually move higher on the **chest wall**, but the hardening of the capsule removes the implant's natural droop, making it look higher. However, nothing is absolute, and on occasion I have seen patients whose implants have actually migrated upward as a result of capsular contracture. In the worst-case scenario, it looks like half a melon on the patient's chest. For most women, this will be considered an unacceptable outcome and require surgical correction.
- ○ **Baker Class IV** capsular contracture refers to a capsule that has become so thick that it has become physically painful. This will obviously require surgical correction and probably the permanent removal or replacement of the implants.

The goal of every implant surgery is to keep the amount of capsular contracture to Class I or II. What are your chances of developing a capsule that becomes a problem? There is no simple statistical number because the risk can be influenced by many factors, including the type of implant used, the placement of the implant in the breast, surgical technique, and, finally, the wild card: genetic predisposition.

There are several factors to consider in terms of the type of implant. The first of these is in regard to the fluid inside of the implant, either silicone gel or saline. For most women, at least in the short term, silicone gel is not an option, but it's worth discussing in the event you do qualify for the gel implants and you are considering trying them (For more on silicone gel implants and who can get them, see Chapters Seven and Eight.). The incidence of Class III or IV capsular contracture increases dramatically with the use of silicone gel. Why this is true remains unclear, but it probably has something to do with trace amounts of the polymer leaching through the implant and into the tissue.

Beyond the choice of filling, implants are available with a textured or smooth surface. The textured surface implants are specifically made to slow or diminish the formation of a capsule, and they are moderately effective. Unfortunately, there is a small cosmetic cost for this decrease in risk, and many women (including most of my patients) continue to opt for the smooth surface shell. The problem is that the textured implant tends to bend a bit, and a ripple or dimple can be seen through the skin in certain positions.

The next factor to consider regarding capsular contracture is the placement of the implant within the breast. Generally, there are two choices, both of which will be discussed at greater length in Chapter Seven. The first option is subglandular and the other is **submuscular**. The chances for Class III or IV capsular contracture are increased with the subglandular placement. For this and other reasons, I do not recommend the subglandular placement, though there are some arguments in its favor.

In my experience, with the above factors figured in, the chance of you having a complicating problem with capsular contracture (Class III or IV) can be summarized as follows:

Silicone gel placed subglandular: 30%-40%
Silicone gel placed submuscular: 15%-17%
Saline implants placed subglandular: 10%-12%
Saline implants placed submuscular: 1%-2%

Most women who look at these figures will see that the clear choice is for a submuscular saline implant. However, every day a certain number of well-informed women make the decision to try the other options above. My fear is that there is another, hopefully small, group of women making these decisions who are not well informed. If you are reading this now, be assured that you are not in that group!

It also must be remembered that statistics are only a guide. If you are in the small group of women who have terrible capsular contracture with textured saline implants placed beneath the muscle, then 1 to 2 percent means nothing to you. For you, as an individual, the number becomes 100 percent! Likewise, I have patients who have silicone gel implants and would never consider changing to saline because, when everything goes well, silicone implants feel like your own breast tissue. In contrast, saline implants always have a discrete feel that alerts anyone feeling them of their unique status. By contrast, I have had many patients tell me that their significant others could not tell that they had silicone implants.

Additionally, the risk percentages are somewhat lower for textured implants. And while these numbers include women who experience complications during surgery, those women that do have complications are at higher risk for capsular contracture. If you develop a hematoma (discussed previously in this chapter) from your surgery, it can be easily dealt with, but unfortunately, the chances of you developing advanced capsular contracture increase slightly.

Finally, some women are apparently genetically predisposed to develop Class III or IV capsules. At the time of writing, there is no test to determine if you fit into this group of women, but with the incredible advances in mapping the human genome we may soon have such a test. Until then, if your mother or sister has had problems with breast implants, you should consider that as an additional risk factor and a sign that you may develop problems as well. Currently, there are studies underway to determine if specific anti-asthma medications can reduce the occurrence of capsular contracture or reverse a previous contracture. Early reports are promising, and anecdotal evidence in my office suggests that these medications may work. See Chapter Ten, "Breast Lift," for further discussion on this topic.

NIPPLE SENSATION

ANOTHER RISK ASSOCIATED with breast enlargement is the loss—or gain—of nipple sensation. A temporary loss of nipple sensation after surgery is common and should not be a cause for alarm. During the normal course of healing and with reduction in swelling, normal sensation should return. However, some women do report a varying degree of loss in nipple sensation. According to a study by the Mentor Corporation, a leading supplier of breast implants, some change in nipple sensation was reported by fifteen percent of the women who had breast enlargement surgery.

There has been some talk about the loss of sensation being caused by the surgeon damaging the nerve during surgery. While this may be the case in some instances, I don't believe that this is normally a problem. The nerve trunk that goes to the nipple is nowhere near any of the usual incision sites for implant placement. Furthermore, while surgical damage to the nerve may explain a loss of sensation, it certainly wouldn't explain a change or even enhancement in sensation. Some women have reported a decrease and others a dramatic increase in sensation that is so intense that it becomes painful, and everything in between. An acquaintance of mine told me the story of a woman he was dating who claimed that prior to implant surgery her nipples were not particular erotically sensitive, but that since surgery her nipples had become such a powerful source of pleasure that she frequently reached orgasm from nipple stimulation alone. Certainly this could not be explained by nerve damage. My theory on all of this, though unproven, is that the implant sometimes causes changes in the transmission of nerve impulses because it exerts a small amount of pressure on the nerve trunk (the part of the nerve that runs between the nerve endings in the skin and the brain) where it passes through the chest wall and into the rib cage. Whatever the reason for these changes, it is a possible risk for you to consider.

LONGEVITY AND RUPTURING OF IMPLANTS

THOUGH THIS IS not a risk factor per se, here is another fact about breast implants that you should definitely consider: The implant is not considered a permanent or "lifetime" device. Your implant *will* eventually leak or rupture. They are designed to last about twenty years and during the course of the first ten years that you have your implants, there is about a 7 percent chance of them rupturing. However, after ten years, the risk of rupture increases each year. In other words, over the course of twenty years, the chance of an implant rupturing is significant. I am often asked when is a good time to exchange the implants or if it's good to change them ten years after surgery. My answer is that these are not tires on your car that require changing before they go bald. With tires, a blowout can be life-threatening, but with implants, a blowout is just an inconvenience. Take a chance and you might be pleasantly surprised to see your implants last fifteen or twenty years.

In the case of saline, the rupturing of the implant is not in any way dangerous. Though it may be alarming when one of your breasts suddenly deflates, the saltwater simply absorbs into the blood stream—which is not at all dangerous, though you may feel an urge to urinate (as if you had drunk a glass of water about the size of your breast implant). The procedure for replacing the ruptured implant is simple, takes only about ten minutes in the office, and requires very little in the way of recovery time or discomfort. Additionally, the replacement implant is provided free of charge by the manufacturer.

The case of a silicone gel implant rupturing is a different story. Under normal circumstances, the silicone gel is too thick to absorb into the body and will, therefore, remain within the capsule formed by the body around the implant. It is likely that you will be unaware of the rupture in this circumstance and there may be no further need of surgery. However, in some cases the silicone gel will leak or break through the capsule—especially in the case of an injury to the breast. Since the gel will not absorb into the body it may flow in odd places and encapsulate there, creating lumps (which are sometimes painful) and hardened areas throughout the chest. It may, in some cases, require extensive surgery to remove all of these silicone gel deposits and, indeed, it may be impossible to get all of it. See Chapters Seven and Eight for more on silicone gel implants.

WHAT ABOUT CANCER?

AT THE TIME of writing, there is absolutely no reason to believe that breast implants have any effect on your chances of getting either breast or any other form of cancer. The longest and most comprehensive studies that have been conducted to date show no increase in cancer for women with breast implants compared with the general population of women who have not had implant surgery. However, if you have a strong family history for breast cancer, you are strongly advised *not* to have breast implants. Why? Because breast implants make breast mammography much more difficult and therefore can make breast cancer harder to detect. As you probably know, the best way to screen for and detect breast cancer early is by having regular **mammograms**. Because the traditional method of taking mammograms will be limited with your implants, additional views must be taken to ensure that your tissue is clear of problems. This will mean that you will be exposed to slightly more X-ray radiation. To be perfectly clear on this issue: Even with the increase in X-ray radiation, it is still *highly* recommended that you continue to receive regular mammograms after implant surgery. Also, the capsule that forms around the implant sometimes has small calcifications, which can be mistaken for cancer, necessitating additional surgery for biopsy and capsule removal. Additionally, ultrasound has been shown to be a helpful method to examine any suspicious solid or cystic lesions.

I should mention that if money is no object (and if you are not claustrophobic) the above problem can be completely resolved by replacing regular mammograms with an MRI outfitted with a breast coil. In this way any potentially dangerous bodies within the breast can be discovered early, without any of the risk associated with X-rays. However, an **MRI** is a costly procedure and it is highly unlikely that your insurance company will pay for even a percentage of it.

Finally, it is essential to give yourself a self-exam for lumps in your breast tissue. Your doctor can quickly show you how to distinguish the implant from your breast tissue. You may even find it simpler to perform the basic self-exam because the implant creates a smooth surface against which to work your fingers.

Implants and Pregnancy

IT HAS been suggested that there might be risks to the children born of mothers with breast implants. While a few studies have been done on the subject, as of yet there does not seem to be any evidence for those fears. That doesn't mean that some sort of other information might not arise in the future but, for the moment at least, there just isn't any reason to believe that there are any problems associated with having children after breast implant surgery.

SILICONE GEL IMPLANTS AND DISEASE

WHAT'S THE DEAL with all of those class action suits from women who say that their breast implants caused all sorts of connective tissue and **autoimmune** diseases? You've probably heard of the horror stories and the multimillion dollar settlements related to breast implants. Over 1.5 million women in the United States have silicone gel implants. There is no doubt that many women who have breast implants are also terribly ill. Many of these women were told in the late 1980s and early 1990s that the source of their illnesses could be traced to their implants. But independent laboratory groups, the **FDA**, and even Congress have conducted studies, and after years of close observation these same women are now being told that the fact that they have breast implants and the fact that they are ill is nothing more than coincidence. They have been victims of both the greed of immoral trial lawyers and the best intentions of ethical trial lawyers, and the victims of the ambiguous nature of scientific inquiry. After all of these many studies, there appears to be absolutely no greater incidence of illness among women with breast implants than with women without implants. A certain number of people will, in the normal course of events, develop terrible diseases such as lupus, rheumatoid arthritis, multiple sclerosis, and fibromyalgia. But there is simply no evidence from the studies that have been conducted that breast implants will increase the occurrence of these diseases.

For women who developed these diseases shortly after obtaining silicone gel implants, and who were perfectly healthy prior to their implant surgeries, this seems ironically unfair.

Furthering their frustration is the fact that some insurance companies deny new policies to any woman who has ever had a ruptured or leaking silicone gel implant, on the grounds that they are more likely to develop certain chronic illnesses. Ironically, insurance companies say there is no danger when implant manufacturers that they insure are sued. Is it possible for the insurance companies to have it both ways?

There is no reason to believe at this time that there is any connection whatsoever between connective tissue or autoimmune diseases and silicone-filled implants. However, as I've discussed, there are other issues associated with silicone gel implants, like rupturing and increased risk of severe capsular contracture, that still make them a poor choice. If safety is a primary concern for you (and it certainly ought to be), you should strongly consider implants with saline. For the present time, in this country, that will be your only option in any case. In the near future, the FDA may expand the use of silicone implants to any patient desiring breast augmentation. At the time of writing, an FDA advisory panel has suggested this change, however, nothing has been determined as of yet. See Chapter Seven and Chapter Eight for options regarding silicone gel implants and the controversy surrounding them.

MINIMIZE YOUR RISKS

STILL INTERESTED IN cosmetic breast surgery? I've presented quite a list of possible problems that you might encounter. If you've read this list of warnings very carefully, you can see that the risks are manageable, but breast surgery is certainly not something that you should enter into frivolously. It is important to understand that there are proactive things that you can do in order to minimize and control the risks involved. Here are a few:

○ **Treat your body well**. Your doctor will likely ask you to try to lose a few pounds on your own if you are seeing him for a reduction. For at least a week prior to your surgery, eat healthy foods and get plenty of sleep. Stress, high blood sugar levels from junk food, and lack of sleep equal a weak immune system to fight infection and a slowed recovery. These dangers can have an avalanche effect and raise the odds of other complications.

○ **If you smoke, quit**. Can I make it any plainer? Your surgeon will (or should) tell you to stop smoking for at least a few weeks prior to surgery. Virtually every risk factor will be reduced if you follow this advice. Among other things, smoking adversely affects circulation and therefore affects blood supply to the very area that needs nutrients, antibodies, and other healing factors to successfully heal. Now, once you've stopped, don't start again. If I'm starting to sound like one of your parents, that's okay. I'm a doctor and a dad, so I won't make any apologies. Quit smoking.

○ **Assess your health**. If you currently have any conditions that might interfere with wound healing or blood clotting, postpone your surgery. If you have a weakened immune system or are taking any immunosuppressive medications, postpone your surgery. If you have any active infection anywhere in your body, postpone your surgery.

○ **Take previous surgery into account**. If you have had previous surgery to your breasts, for example, or if you are seeking an improvement after previous cosmetic work or an improved appearance after an injury, you might have a reduced blood supply to your breasts. In this event you should seriously consider not having cosmetic breast surgery that might damage the remaining blood supply. Your doctor will certainly discuss this possibility with you if you fall into this group. Find a surgeon who specializes in revision work, and be sure that your doctor asks for and reviews the old operative because this will provide your physician with critical information necessary to determine which procedure is right for you.

○ **Become an informed consumer**. You should know exactly what to expect from your particular procedure. You should know what is normal and what is not normal during recovery, what warning signs to look out for, and what they mean.

○ **Plan for your surgery**. Make sure that you have set up your home and your life before your surgery so that you will have an easy and stress-free surgery and recovery. In other words, if you have a two-year-old child and no childcare options, you should postpone your surgery. You can always do it down the road.

○ **Communicate with your surgeon**. Make sure that your surgeon is someone you can trust in the event that things go wrong. Making smart choices is key to success in anything, and surgery is certainly no exception. If you feel that you don't communicate well with your surgeon, postpone your surgery. Perhaps the main factor in minimizing all of the other risk factors is finding the right surgeon and, in the next chapter, this is discussed in detail.

THE REWARDS

BESIDES HAVING REALLY great-looking breasts, there are some clear benefits to having cosmetic breast surgery. While some may be obvious to you, others may not.

The most definitive benefit of cosmetic breast surgery is for patients who have chosen surgery for more than merely cosmetic reasons. If you are having a breast reduction to ease the symptoms of back and neck pain from breasts that are simply too large and heavy for your frame, you will almost certainly obtain relief. For women in this category surgery is truly a case of getting your life back. Also, if you are a woman who has had or is going to have mastectomy surgery and you are considering reconstruction, an overwhelming number of studies show that women who have reconstruction are many times less likely to develop depression and other psychological complications as a result of this difficult process.

It should be obvious if you are choosing to have breast surgery purely for cosmetic reasons that it will positively impact your self-esteem. What may not be obvious is the powerful effect that a boost in self-esteem can have on your life. For example, women who have had cosmetic breast surgery who were previously overweight very frequently begin to successfully lose weight after their surgery. This can only be attributed to a boost in self-esteem, and it seems logical as well. If you like your body, you are more likely to want to do something nice for it, and that includes things like eating healthy foods and exercising regularly. The people who continually fail to stay with a diet or exercise program tend to be people with a negative body image. It's hard to do something that's good for your body when your body is your enemy.

There is plenty of clinical evidence that a boost in self-esteem has powerful benefits for a person's personal and emotional life. That has certainly been my observation with my own patients and it is incredibly gratifying. A particularly powerful example of how a change in your self image can dramatically change your life was brought to me by one of my own patients. When Jenny first came to my office, she was engaged to be married the following year. After many, many years of thinking about it, she decided it was time to finally have the breast enlargement that she always wanted, as a wedding present to herself. Like many of my patients, Jenny felt boyish because she was tall and had very small breasts. For her wedding, she wanted to feel feminine and she had a particular longing for looking a certain way in her wedding dress. She had a very simple procedure with smooth saline implants and a very brief and easy recovery period, so after a few months I didn't see much of her.

However, since she was very pleased with her new breasts, I was not at all surprised when a year later a woman came in to my office who said that I was recommended by her good friend Jenny. I did a brief calculation in my head and realized that Jenny must now be married, so I asked her friend how the wedding went.

"Wedding? Oh, no," said her friend. "Jenny dumped that guy. He was never right for her, but we could never convince her of that because she had such a low opinion of herself."

I couldn't believe my ears. Her friend went on to say that after her surgery, Jenny had become much more social and began meeting many more men who wanted to date her. She quickly realized that she wasn't dependent on this guy; that she had options. She began to realize that what her friends had been telling her all along was true. Settling for this guy would be a terrible mistake. The last I heard, Jenny was once again engaged, this time to a man who is a great catch.

I hope that nobody who reads this story thinks that cosmetic breast surgery is like some kind of fairy-tale or glass slipper that will cause Prince Charming to come running. I don't believe for an instant that Jenny attracted more men because she had larger breasts. The real point of this story, and the thing that I hope you take from it, is what breast surgery *can* do is make you feel better about yourself. And feeling better about yourself can be a very powerful force in your life, sometimes in ways that you don't expect.

5
Choosing a Surgeon
Your Biggest Decision

Y OUR RELATIONSHIP WITH your surgeon neither begins nor ends with your surgery. It would be a mistake to think that it's all right to not get along well with your surgeon as long as he or she has an excellent reputation and is known for doing beautiful work. You should consider both as necessary requirements in choosing your doctor. If you do not have a good relationship with your surgeon—if you do not feel completely comfortable during your conversations together—there is an excellent chance that you will not be satisfied with your final results. Furthermore, you must consider that even when things go perfectly, your relationship with your surgeon is a long-term venture, with follow-up visits and examinations that may last for many years. If things don't go perfectly well you may end up spending much more time with this person than you had originally anticipated.

This chapter will outline the key parameters you should always refer to when choosing your plastic surgeon (or any doctor, for that matter). Credentials are always an ideal starting point for all physicians. However, any wonderful residency program has its share of duds. Therefore, getting references from your friends and physicians will certainly help to narrow down the list of candidates. Meeting with the surgeon, examining his or her portfolio, talking to his or her patients, and developing a comfortable rapport are essential to making the correct choice

HOW DO YOU START?

THE IDEAL STARTING point is to assemble a list of names of surgeons in your area who might be of interest to you. Some physicians may be culled from websites, professional organizations, the phone book, or advertisements in your local paper. Although many of these physicians may be excellent, be careful that they satisfy all the other criteria elucidated in this chapter. Picking a name from the phone book, without a more thorough investigation, is a great way to look for trouble. You can get names from friends who have had plastic surgery and are *pleased* with their results. You can also get names from your personal physician, who may have a relationship with a local plastic surgeon. Doctors are often very careful to refer their patients to reputable specialists, because a bad referral reflects poorly on their own skills as a doctor.

Once you have assembled the list of surgeons, cut it down to a manageable number of physicians based on the other criteria discussed below. Please don't use cost as a limiting criteria. The cheapest surgeon may be good, but he may not. Why is he the cheapest? The cost of corrections may easily wipe out any initial cost savings.

▷ What Are the Surgeon's Credentials?

You should find out about board certifications, surgical experience, and hospitals that have granted your doctor surgical privileges. If your doctor is board certified, ask by which board or boards. All plastic surgeons should be certified by the **American Board of Plastic Surgery**. There is no other board sanctioned to certify plastic surgeons. There are many fancy sounding board certifications but this is the only one that counts! If you have gotten to this point, and have a list of surgeons who are board certified, your work is only partly over. Even with the qualifications necessary for board certification, by no means does this rule out mediocre or even poor surgeons.

As for surgical experience, it is certainly worthwhile to find out how many surgeries your doctor has performed that are *similar to your specific procedure*. You don't want to be anyone's practice session. Conversely, some surgeons have generated large practices by advertising or through other means and by necessity must perform many procedures to generate income. For these physicians the patient is a number; individuality and expertise are lost. Be sure that your physician takes the time to understand you and your desires. You should also ask your prospective surgeon about hospital affiliations and surgical privileges. Because hospitals have their own reputations to protect and state regulations to follow, they are also careful about the doctors to whom they grant surgical privileges.

▷ Play Sherlock Holmes

Once you have found out about your prospective surgeon's credentials, you are off to a good start. If you want to do a little private detective work on your own, many states keep track of patient complaints lodged against doctors and you can easily access that information on the Internet. Try typing "complaints," "doctors," and "state," ("state" means the state in which the doctor is practicing) in the search line of your favorite Internet search engine and you will probably find the information on the first page of results. For example, searching "complaints, doctors, New York" on Google gave me the New York State Department of Health's Professional Misconduct and Physician Discipline page as the first result. This is the organization in New York State responsible for investigating complaints against doctors and it provides a list of physicians who have been disciplined.

Before my colleagues lynch me, I must explain that the mere presence of complaints against a surgeon does not necessarily mean that you have located a bad surgeon. Complaints are fairly normal in the course of doing business with the public. There will always be patients who will lodge a complaint against a doctor regardless of the quality of service rendered and there are many truly excellent surgeons who have had such complaints filed. Be particularly suspicious of a pattern of a particular problem, but even if a doctor had only a single complaint filed, it would certainly behoove you to discuss this with him or her. If the doctor cannot explain the complaint to your satisfaction, you may very well have uncovered a problem.

▷ References

Many women find their surgeon through friends who have provided recommendations. Friends are the very best references because they are people that you know and trust and, therefore, you are likely to get a lot of useful and unbiased information from them. If you find a surgeon from a website, a professional organization, or the phone book, ask for references and then contact them. You would assume that any references given by the surgeon's office are for patients that they are certain will have no complaints, but it's amazing how frequently checking such references can provide useful information. A surgeon who does not generally have good doctor-patient relationships won't know with certainty what those patients are saying.

When checking a surgeon's references, always ask specific questions about the patient's procedure. Make an attempt to verify that the reference is for real. If you truly are interested in choosing a physician, try to meet the reference in person to be certain that the outcome is what you are hoping for.

▷ The Portfolio

Now that basics are out of the way, let's get into the real work of finding the right surgeon for you. It's time to look at the doctor's portfolio. Every serious plastic surgeon has a book of before-and-after photos of their patients. You need to take a look at these. Don't be wowed by a bunch of perfect little breasts that have become perfect larger breasts. Any surgeon can make an already good-looking breast look good. This is not enough. (Obviously the exception here is if you are a woman with perfect *little* breasts who desires perfect *larger* breasts—these photos then apply directly to your situation.) Generally, you want to find a "before" picture that shows a patient with breasts that look like your own, has your same set of problems, and similar or identical goals. If you like the "after" photo, you are definitely on the right track. This surgeon just might be for you.

You might want to point out the particular before-and-after photos that seem to deal with your situation and ask the surgeon what technique he or she used on this particular woman and whether or not you would be a good candidate for the same procedure. It is possible that to your untrained eye the woman in the picture has the same problem that you have, but the surgeon may point out some critical differences that will require you to have a very different procedure. If this is the case, you need to see photos of women who have had that procedure. If you still like what you are seeing, you will probably feel pretty good about this doctor. But we're not finished yet.

YOUR RELATIONSHIP WITH YOUR SURGEON

BY NOW WE may have determined that the doctor in question has the right technical background and skills. The next questions are: Can you feel comfortable with this person and talk to him or her effectively? It is very important that when you speak you feel that your doctor listens to you and understands what you are saying. Since surgery is largely irreversible, it's a good idea to get things right the first time. Your surgeon must understand your goal exactly and be able to tell you what your different options are in trying to achieve that goal. If you feel that the doctor understands you, the next obvious question is, do you understand this surgeon? Do you like what he or she says? Do his or her suggestions make sense to you? Rely on your instincts. If you feel like a surgeon's suggestions for cosmetic procedures don't match your goals, you are probably right. Don't let some doctor try to convince you to put a square peg in a round hole. But if you speak to several surgeons and they all seem to think your goals are unrealistic, then perhaps you need to re-evaluate your own expectations and requirements. For example, if you really want a breast lift and reshaping without any visible scars, you will not like your options and no credible surgeon is going to be able to satisfy you.

It's important not to choose a doctor based on everything going right. On the contrary, you must base your decision on every conceivable thing going wrong. In the gravest extreme, is this the surgeon you trust to stand beside you? In the worst-case scenario, do you feel comfortable placing your health in this person's hands? You want more than a talented plastic surgeon;

you want a good doctor who cares about your health and well-being.

A good indicator of whether a surgeon is a good one is during the initial exam. A surgeon who merely takes measurements of your breasts is obviously only prepared to care for your breasts and you should consider this a warning sign. If an assistant examines you at the initial visit, you can be certain that the surgeon knows little about you. Furthermore, he or she is relying on someone else's judgment to determine your unique situation and surgical needs. A proper and thorough examination of your overall health shows professional responsibility and is a good sign. You shouldn't put the appearance of your breasts over your health and your plastic surgeon shouldn't either. If your doctor drives you crazy about quitting smoking or eating healthy foods, you've probably found someone whom you can trust.

Cost-Cutting Surgeons in Other Countries Are Probably Not Worth It

A SERIOUS new phenomenon has recently cropped up that I think deserves some attention. Several women have come to my office with post-surgical problems as a result of undergoing cosmetic breast surgery in another country. These patients elected to undergo surgery elsewhere because of the expected cost savings. This choice violates many of the suggestions I have made up to this point. Be very wary of choosing to have surgery in another country. What do you know about this physician? Is he or she board certified? What criteria regulate the surgical facilities? What happens if you develop a problem? Are you going to fly back to Costa Rica, for weekly visits? Clearly, the expected cost savings can be extremely expensive to you in the long run.

ASK QUESTIONS

ONCE YOU'VE FOUND a surgeon who you feel is technically capable of performing the procedure you desire, who you can communicate with, and who you trust, don't be afraid to ask any question. One of the paramount rules of managing the risks inherent in your surgery is becoming an educated consumer. Your doctor should welcome these questions. Don't be afraid to bring a list.

One of my recent patients had considered cosmetic breast surgery for a number of years before taking the leap. She had decided to wait until after she had her kids because she had read that childbirth and breast-feeding can make cosmetically enhanced breasts just as saggy as natural breasts and she didn't want to have surgery twice. She spoke to the doctors who knew her health history the best—her family doctor and to her gynecologist—to assess the risks to her health. Then she asked some of her friends for references and recommendations and visited three other plastic surgeons before she showed up in my office. When she arrived for her initial consultation with me, she brought a long laundry list of questions. I'll be honest; I liked all of this careful preparation so much that I immediately ignored the fact that her husband was also really excited about her upcoming breast enlargement.

Breast-Feeding
Can You? Should You?

HE RISKS TO BREAST-FEEDING associated with cosmetic breast surgery vary widely from procedure to procedure. However, with every procedure there is at least some degree of risk that you might not be able to breast-feed post-surgery. So if breast-feeding is extremely important to you as an individual, you should put off your surgery until after your children are weaned. Additionally, breast-feeding is very likely to change the shape of your breasts, so if you are planning to become pregnant in the near future and you would prefer to nurse your child, it might be a waste of your time and money to have your surgery now. If, on the other hand, you are young, unmarried, thinking of having kids ten years down the road, would prefer nursing but would not be overly upset by having to bottle-feed, the breast-feeding issue should not be a big concern for you. This chapter will explain the individual considerations of the major cosmetic breasts procedures and breast-feeding. Since breast augmentation is the most common, I'll start there.

BREAST-FEEDING AND AUGMENTATION

A SINGLE STUDY suggests that 64 percent of women with implants could not breast-feed, compared to 7 percent of women without implants. These figures may be somewhat deceiving, however, because most women who desire breast augmentation have small breasts and would find it more difficult to breast-feed had they not had surgery at all. Furthermore, patients that lose nipple sensation are advised to avoid breast-feeding. Generally speaking, there is no reason that you should not be able to breast-feed after implant surgery. As mentioned in Chapter Four on the risks and rewards of silicone gel implants, there have been fears that silicone may leach into the breast milk and negatively affect your baby. At the time of writing, there is no proven evidence of this. Since silicone gel implants are, for the time being, difficult to obtain anyway, there shouldn't be any cause for worry. A study measuring silicon (one component in silicone) levels in breast milk did not find any significant amount in the breast milk of patients with breast implants. In a very small number of cases where serious surgical complications arise, it is possible that damage might occur to the ducts that carry the milk from the milk glands to the nipples, but this is very uncommon.

If you're interested in having a lift or reduction, your doctor can give you an accurate idea of the risk entailed with your particular procedure. However, note that some procedures, notably **free-nipple procedures** (where the nipple is removed completely from the underlying tissue), involve cutting the milk ducts and remove the option of using a breast pump. The only remaining option would be bottle feeding, using formula.

One simple and common cosmetic procedure that many women seek is to correct "innie" nipples. In these women, instead of protruding in the natural manner, their nipples pucker inward. This is caused by shorter than normal milk ducts and the surgical solution to the problem is to simply cut the ducts. If you are considering having children, you should be advised that this procedure rules out any chance of breast-feeding.

The larger concern has to do with the loss of nipple sensation, which could potentially be caused by any type of cosmetic breast surgery. Loss of nipple sensation effectively prevents you from nursing at the breast because you will be unaware of what would otherwise be painful behavior from the infant. Normally if there is any pain, the mother temporarily pulls the child away from the nipple. Without sensation, the baby could damage the nipple or areola. This, in turn, could cause a localized infection called **mastitis**. Most doctors agree that the risk of mastitis is too great to persevere with breast-feeding if you have any loss of nipple sensation.

The good news is that there is no reason that you can't use a breast pump to obtain natural breast milk for your baby. Even with no nipple sensation at all, you can save yourself the risk of mastitis and still give your baby the full benefits and nutrients of your breast milk by using a pump. However, if your reasons for wanting to breast-feed have more to do with the intimate feelings of bonding with your child in this special way, the loss of nipple sensation will be a much bigger issue.

If you are considering having children at some time in the future, but are very eager to have cosmetic breast surgery immediately, you must consider how important breast-feeding is to you. If you are married, how important is it to your spouse who, as an equal partner in the parenting of the child, should have at least some say in the matter? Many children around the world have been exclusively bottle fed on formula and have grown up perfectly healthy and happy. If breast milk for your baby is important, decide if pumping is a good option for you. This will open up a very large range of surgical options. Discuss the issue with your doctor to determine if you can achieve the results you desire without a great risk of damaging the milk ducts. If your chosen procedure will require the severing of the milk ducts, or if it is essential to you that your baby receives milk directly from your breast, you have a difficult decision ahead of you: You must decide between delaying your surgery and compromising your desires regarding breast-feeding.

Breast Enlargement

*Getting It Right
the First Time*

THE MOST COMMONLY requested cosmetic surgical procedure for women in America is the breast augmentation, or enlargement. So odds are if you're reading this book, then you are particularly interested in this chapter. All breast enlargements involve the placement of some kind of implant within the breast, but the type of implant, where it is placed within the breast, and how it gets there can vary widely, so there are many factors to consider before going ahead with your surgery.

This chapter will discuss breast augmentation in depth. It will explain the difference between different implant sizes and shapes. After reading this chapter, you will understand the individual risks and benefits of each type of enlargement procedure (not all procedures are the same!). I will also show you how to determine what breast implant size is correct for you. Don't leave these important decisions up to your surgeon. This is a personal decision, and only *your* desires should come into play.

SOME WORDS ABOUT SILICONE

ONE QUESTION MANY women ask is what exactly is a silicone gel implant, and if the studies don't show them to be harmful, why can't I get them? Let's start at the beginning. Silicone is a polymer (complex chemical) that is based on silicon, a basic element found in nature and one of the most common basic chemicals in the world. Beach sand and glass are both made of silicon. The shell or outer bag of all breast implants is made from silicone. Many other materials have been tried and tested for this purpose, but silicone has been found to be the best and the safest of all known alternatives. Even though all breast implants have a shell made of silicone, they may be filled with either saline or another form of silicone called silicone gel.

Some women want to get implants filled with silicone gel because they feel softer and more natural than saline. In fact, silicone gel feels almost exactly like natural, firm breast tissue. However, at this time, silicone implants are in clinical trials in this country and are limited to patients who fall into specific categories. This is primarily due to the enormous class action lawsuits that began twenty years ago. Even though current research shows that silicone gel is safe for most women, the FDA has not approved its use in implants. As I have mentioned previously, the FDA advisory panel has recommended that silicone implants be made available to all patients. As of January 2004, this recommendation has been taken under advisement and it may have become law by the time you read this. You can go to the implant manufacturers' websites— www.inamed.com and www.mentorcorp.com—to check on the current status of silicone implants. While most of the science shows that these implants are safe, I still advise my patients against them because the risk of serious capsular contracture (Baker Class III or IV) is dramatically higher with silicone gel. However, no breast implants, including those filled with silicone gel, have been shown to cause cancer or any other connective tissue disease.

If you are determined to have silicone gel implants, there are loopholes in the law that you may want to seek out. The first step is to become part of the FDA's study on silicone gel implants, for which there are strict standards. To be eligible, you need to fall into one of four categories:

1. Women who are getting breast reconstruction after mastectomy may obtain silicone gel implants.
2. Women who have previously had or currently have silicone gel implants are also automatically eligible.
3. Women who have a medical necessity for implant surgery. It is in this category that some unethical surgeons have obtained permission for their patients to enter the study. These surgeons risk both their medical license and the health of their patients.
4. In some cases, women who are having a breast augmentation in addition to a lift will qualify for silicone. There are also women who skirt the FDA regulations by going overseas to have their breast augmentation. Silicone gel implants are still legal in Europe and may be obtained by American citizens who are willing to pay the cost and take the associated risks.

For more on silicone gel implants, please read the next chapter. I will devote the rest of this chapter to saline-filled implants because they are legal in all cases, they are safer, and they have a much lower risk of capsular contracture and, consequently, patient dissatisfaction.

Implants and Leakage

> **REMEMBER:** Implants are not lifetime devices; they will leak eventually. Most leakage occurs fifteen to twenty-five years after placement, but since they are filled with saltwater, it is perfectly safe. The procedure to replace a leaking implant is simple, fast, and painless. And most manufacturers of implants will give you free replacement implants of the same size for life.

TEXTURES AND SHAPES

WHAT TYPES OF saline implants are available? First, as I briefly discussed in Chapter Four, there are textured and smooth implants. Textured implants are marginally safer in terms of capsule formation but are cosmetically inferior because of their tendency to form a visible ripple in the breast. I generally recommend smooth implants because the gain in safety with textured implants is not great enough to justify the higher aesthetic price, but the choice ultimately rests with the patient.

Implants also come in different shapes. The most common implant is the plain, round implant. For women who desire more forward projection in their breasts, there is also a type of implant called the **high profile breast implant**, which is

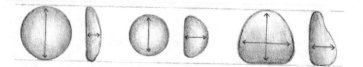

There are three types of implants: Round implants (left) have two dimensions: width and height/projection; a special round implant, known as a high profile implant (middle), is narrower than the normal profile implant with the added benefit of greater projection; anatomic implants (right) are designed to create a teardrop shape. They present an asymmetrical profile (height and width are not equal).

slightly more conical in the front and slightly narrower in width. Also available are the anatomical or teardrop-shaped implants that are designed to create a more natural-looking breast.

The high profile implant gives excellent results for women who wish to have their breasts project farther in front of their chests. This type of implant is excellent for patients who have narrow chests but still desire dramatic projection. A round implant that would give this patient the desired projection might be too wide to accommodate her narrow chest. The limitation of high profile implants is that some women find them too narrow for their chest wall, yielding an extremely wide cleavage; or, for some patients with a narrow chest wall, the resultant cleavage is extreme and unnatural in appearance. This is a situation that your surgeon will advise you about if you are considering the high profile implant.

Another option for women with narrow chests that yields very similar results is to slightly overfill conventional round implants. Overfilling tends to narrow the dimension of the implant while increasing projection. Many surgeons advise their patients to have overfilled implants as a matter of routine. They suggest that overfilling implants may reduce rippling and sagging. The manufacturers of implants do not recommend this procedure, as it may decrease the lifespan of the implant and cause it to break down sooner, and it may also increase the appearance of ripples, in contrast to your surgeon's advice. However, for a woman who wants the look of a high-profile implant whose body is not narrow enough to accommodate it, overfilling does not seem to present any safety hazard.

Anatomical implants are teardrop shaped and therefore have an axis. This means that the height and width of the implants are different. Two correctly placed implants will look identical, but if either implant is rotated slightly in either direction, without moving or rotating the other, noticeable asymmetry will result. Figure five shows how a rotated implant can distort a

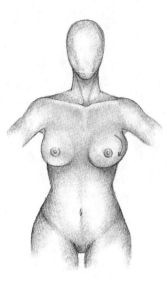

Anatomical implants have an asymmetrical profile. Any rotation of either implant not duplicated on the other side will be noticeable.

breast's shape. Notice the asymmetry caused by one of the teardropped-shaped implants rotating sideways. This risk must be taken into account if you are considering the anatomical implant. I personally think that a very natural looking result can be achieved without having to risk using an anatomical implant that might shift its position. Recent studies suggest that round implants actually assume a teardrop shape within the body about six months after they have been placed, thus eliminating any benefits of the teardrop implant.

The last type of available implant is the **postoperatively adjustable implant**. Most implants have a self-sealing valve on the front that is used to fill the implant during surgery, once the surgeon has placed it within the breast. A postoperatively adjustable implant has a special valve that allows saline to be added or removed *after* the surgery is completed. The wonderful thing about this is that it allows you to see exactly what your breasts look like at a particular size and then add or remove volume until your breasts are exactly the way you had envisioned them. While this is really a great idea, in practice there are some shortcomings to the adjustable implant. Many women do not like having the small valve used for adjusting the saline volume poking through their skin after surgery. Ultimately, once the implant has been filled to the satisfaction of the patient, the valve and tube are removed, but many patients simply don't like the idea of having it there at all after surgery—or the idea of the second minor surgery required to remove the valve. Still, many women choose to have them because figuring out the correct size for implants can be such a difficult and frustrating process.

DO YOU WANT REGULAR, LARGE, OR SUPER-SIZE?

IT IS SIMPLY impossible to know exactly what your breasts will look like after implant surgery. You've seen certain breasts that you may think look great, but what will they look like on your body? Women are basically divided into three groups in terms of how large they want their breasts to be.

The first group is looking for just a subtle change. Their goal is for their breasts to be larger, fuller, and prettier but without anyone necessarily noticing that they've had surgery. They want the difference to be just large enough to show, but not enough to raise eyebrows at the office. This patient is frequently a woman with smallish breasts who has had children and basically wants to restore a bit of fullness to her breasts that has been lost—and perhaps just a bit more.

The second group of women is looking for a significant change. They want to go as large as they possibly can while still looking natural. The idea is that anyone who knows them will certainly recognize that they have had a breast augmentation, but anybody who they meet afterward will not be able to tell.

This is probably the largest group of patients I see. While I am confident in my work in terms of making the finished breast look very natural, the challenge is knowing what the maximum enlargement can be before the woman's breasts simply look too large to be natural. Considerations of tissue, body size, proportion, and size of the ribcage all come into play.

The last group is made up of women who want their breasts to look blatantly fake. They don't care about looking natural or have issues of proportion, they just want the largest breasts that they can comfortably and safely carry.

Every woman has had the experience of going to a hairstylist to try something new and leaving disappointed. Sometimes this is because the woman didn't communicate well with the stylist and, so, ended up with something different than she had wanted. Sometimes it's because the style she had in mind looked great in the magazine or on her friend, but didn't look the way they thought it would with her own hair and with their face. This same thing can happen with cosmetic breast surgery. But unlike hair color or cut, it is much more complicated to change if you don't like it. So it is very important that you are as certain as possible that you know what you want before you have your surgery.

Choose Your Breasts Carefully

I HAD a patient who was referred to me by her sister. Since she had a very similar frame as her sister, she had an excellent idea of what she would look like with implants of the same size. So we both had a great deal of confidence in her decision when she said that she wanted her breasts similar to, but just a little bit smaller than her sister's. However, not long after her surgery, she changed her mind. She wanted her breasts to be slightly larger than her sister's. So, we did a second surgery and replaced her implants with a larger size. Although a second surgery to replace implants is a far easier and less painful procedure, this procedure was still surgery and not without risk. And if someone in this patient's position can make a mistake about what she wanted, even with a nearly perfect example to compare herself with, you can imagine that it really is quite challenging to determine exactly what you want. The main thing is to keep in mind that this is a long-term decision, so don't rush it.

So how do you decide what size is right for you? There are a few things that will help you decide. Many women like to bring in photographs of topless women who have what they consider the right size. Certainly there is no shortage of these kinds of photographs; there seems to be a virtually limitless number on the Internet and in magazines. Some women talk to friends and others who have breasts that they think are the right size. This can be tricky, as the patient gets caught up in cup size or ccs (the amount of saline in an implant is measured in ccs-cubic centimeters). It's a good idea to bring your surgeon a photo of someone with your ideal breasts and ask, "How large an implant would I need, considering my body as it is, to achieve a look similar to her?" This will help you arrive at a ballpark figure.

Using cup size as a guideline is difficult because it does not take into account the differences in body type and size. A C-cup may look perfect on one woman and be far too large or too small on another. Your overall shape and height as well as the size of your rib cage, waist, hips, shoulders, and length of your torso will all dramatically change how a given cup size will look on you.

The problem is further aggravated when trying to use ccs or implant size as a guideline. Not only do all of the problems associated with cup-size exist, but every woman has a different amount of breast tissue to start out with. Thus a woman who already has fairly large breasts will obtain much larger breasts with the same size implant as a woman who started out with very small breasts. Even small differences in the amount of breast tissue and the way the tissue is distributed can yield a very different result.

There is an excellent technique called the **rice test**, that you can try at home even before you speak to a doctor. You will need some plastic sandwich bags, a measuring cup, and a package of dry, uncooked rice. Pour some rice into two bags, squeeze out all the air, and tie the bags with twist-ties. Then tuck the bags of rice into your bra. Flatten the rice out to assume the shape of your breasts and throw a shirt on and take a look at the size of your breasts. Continue to add or remove rice from the bags until you find the size that you think looks right on you. Then simply measure the rice in the measuring cup. Most measuring cups sold today include a scale for measuring in cc or ml (milliliter, which are the same as cc). Don't be surprised if you have a different volume of rice for the left and right breasts, nobody is perfectly symmetrical. It is important to try this test with a bathing suit, T-shirt, blouse, and sweater. As the type of clothing changes, so will your appearance. Small implants will perhaps be satisfactory for the summer in a bikini and T-shirt, but unacceptable in a sweater. Many patients tell me that they want to fill out a sweater, but when they try the appropriate rice implant with a bathing suit, they realize that the implants are too big. Sizing the correct implant for you is the great balancing act of the seasons. I often hear from patients in the winter, wishing they had larger implants, but when they return in the summer their concerns have lessened.

I recommend that you repeat the rice procedure every night for a week, starting with the amount that you thought was right the night before. You will probably find that as your eye gets used to the new look you will want to go with a slightly larger volume, though smaller is also possible. Once you have found a volume that you are happy with, you will be in an excellent position to discuss with your surgeon the size of the implant that you would like.

Based on your surgeon's examination, you should be ready to take the next step and talk about placement and procedure. The only snag might be that if you want dramatically larger breasts, it may be possible that what you want is bigger than you can physically accommodate. Some women, particularly young, thin women, simply don't have enough skin to stretch over the size of the implant that they desire. In such a case you might have to settle for something smaller, at least for the short term. Over time your skin and tissue may stretch to accommodate the extra volume in your breasts and you will then be able to switch up to a larger size implant. This two-step procedure is not uncommon and in some cases is the only viable option if you want dramatically larger breasts.

LOCATION, LOCATION, LOCATION

THE NEXT ISSUE is where the implant will be placed within your breast. There are only two options: subglandular and submuscular. In the subglandular placement, the implant sits between the milk-producing gland of the breast and the pectoral muscle that lies beneath the gland. With submuscular placement, the implant is actually buried beneath the muscle along the chest wall. Most surgeons recommend and most women opt for submuscular placement.

Subglandular surgery is easier, the recovery is quicker, and it is substantially less painful (indeed, sometimes it is completely painless). So why isn't it the more popular placement? The first reason is that, as mentioned in the chapter on risks and rewards, the chances of you developing problems with capsular contracture are far greater with an implant that is placed in

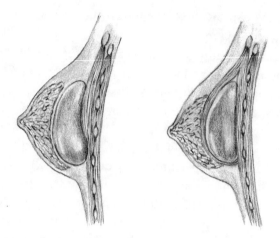

Side view cutaway of implants placed in front of the pectoralis major muscle (subglandular) on the left and behind the same muscle (submuscular) on the right. The submuscular placement creates a more natural shape to the implant.

the subglandular position. Since this is (and should be) a paramount concern for most women having breast augmentations, this is reason enough. The other reason is that submuscular placement usually looks and feels much more natural because the firm muscle tissue does a better job of hiding the outline of the implant.

Still, there are women who simply don't want the additional pain and recovery time of the submuscular placement. Often they have friends who have subglandular implants and they like the way their friends' breasts look. But since this is a long-term decision, I always recommend the submuscular placement.

SURGICAL PROCEDURES AND SCARS

OVER THE YEARS, surgeons have developed all sorts of ways to get the implant into the breast. The two goals of every surgical technique are to place the implant correctly into position in the safest and surest manner and to minimize or hide the scars from the incision sites as much as possible. Based on these two goals each technique has its benefits and its problems and, sometimes, one goal must be sacrificed for the other.

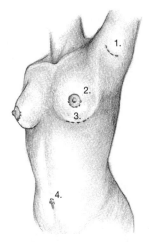

Each of the four different breast implant incisions are depicted with broken lines: 1) Trans-axillary (armpit) 2) Periareolar (around the nipple) 3) Inframammary (under the breast) 4) Trans-umbilical (through the belly button).

An extreme example of this sacrificing is the **trans-umbilical endoscopic augmentation (TUBA) technique** (see illustration on page 79). Using this technique a surgeon can virtually eliminate any visible scars. This amazing feat is accomplished by inserting the implants through an incision in the belly button. This requires the surgeon to essentially dig a tunnel beneath the skin from the navel to the chest and then, using an **endoscope**, create the pocket for the implant, expand the tissue, and insert and fill the implant. The endoscope is a tiny camera that sits at the end of a long tube that allows surgeons to peer inside the body and do surgery by "remote control" in areas that they could not otherwise see. If it sounds difficult, that's because it is. When everything goes perfectly, it is possible to have breast implant surgery with no visible scar at all since the only cut is made inside the belly button.

However, the major manufacturers of implants strongly caution all women *against* this procedure. First, it is very difficult to precisely create the pocket in which the implant will be placed using an endoscope in such a position. Instead of carefully creating the pocket with standard surgical instruments, the surgeon must rely on a **tissue expander**, which is a spring-operated device at the end of a flexible rod that expands above the muscle to open a space for the implant. In order to use the tissue expander, the surgeon must temporarily remove the endoscope. This is a very imprecise method and frequently leads to asymmetry or worse. Second, in order to tunnel from the belly button to the breasts, the surgeon must cut through the **inframammary fold**—the strong tissue at the base of the breasts that attaches to the chest wall. This can create problems that are very difficult to repair, including asymmetry, lowering of the inframammary fold, and resultant implant ptosis (sagging). And finally, everything must be done indirectly while watching though the endoscope. This complicates everything from the basic insertion of the implant to controlling bleeding and minimizing the occurrence of hematomas or other complications. I believe that at this time the risks associated with this procedure are simply unacceptable and I have avoided offering it to my own patients. Unfortunately, it is gaining in popularity and many of the women who come to me to fix prior bad surgery have undergone this basically unstudied procedure.

The other extreme is the **inframammary technique**. This involves making the incision at the bottom of the breast where it attaches to the chest. This is an area that is hidden by the breast on most women (the exception being women with very small breasts) when they are standing up. However, the scar usually becomes visible when you lie down. This direct technique

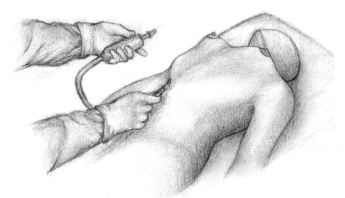

Depiction of a trans-umbilical breast augmentation (TUBA). The surgeon places an instrument through the belly button, under the skin toward the breast. A pocket is blindly created under the breast and then the implant is passed through the tunnel.

is very simple to perform, consistently yields excellent results, shortens recovery time, and reduces the chances of complications. For women with large breasts and women with skin that normally scars very faintly, or for women who don't mind the appearance of the scar when lying down topless, this remains an excellent and conservative surgical choice. However for some women, the scar may widen as a result of the stress of breast expansion and may also migrate onto the breast as the lower pole of the breast is expanded.

A very popular technique right now is the **trans-axillary technique**, where the surgeon goes in through the underarm. The reason for its popularity is that many women like the idea of having their scar away from their breasts—after all it's their breasts that they are trying to make more beautiful. The axillary technique, like the TUBA technique, requires the surgeon to create a pocket for the implant and to control bleeding by remote viewing with an endoscope. Therefore even though many women do achieve excellent results with this procedure and it is fairly common, it is still a more difficult and riskier procedure (though in no way as risky as the TUBA). With this technique, it is very difficult to re-adjust the amount of saline in the implant once it is filled and the fill-tube is removed. If you develop a hematoma or bleeding occurs, your surgeon may have to perform an additional surgery to fix the problem—and that will most likely mean an additional scar on the breast in addition to the underarm site. It is quite difficult to control bleeding through the axillary incision. Another common problem with the axillary procedure is that because the surgeon is creating the pocket from the outer, upper-half of the muscle, closest to the armpit, some women have a problem with the implant slipping to the side. Specifically, when they lie on their backs, the implant has a tendency to slip down into their armpit. This can be disconcerting to say the least. And, finally, while the axillary procedure offers the benefit of having no scar on the breast itself, the scar that does result is the only one of the various techniques that can be visible even in clothing. If you wear a halter top, tank top, or swimsuit, the scar may be clearly visible when you raise your arm.

The last method that I will discuss is the **periareolar technique**. It is the technique that I prefer and the one I think makes the most sense. In the periareolar procedure the surgeon makes the incision around the edge of the nipple. Because there is a natural border in color between the areola and the rest of the breast, the scar is usually very well concealed. Certainly, it cannot be seen in a swimsuit or any other clothing, and frequently it will go unnoticed when you are topless, except when viewed very closely. The periareolar incision is almost as simple as the inframammary incision and allows the surgeon a great deal of control in terms of precise pocket placement, adjusting the fill of the implant, and safety issues, like controlling bleeding.

Some women fear that there is a greater incidence of loss of nipple sensation with the periareolar technique. This sounds logical because if you are cutting closer to the nipple, you are more likely to damage its nerves but, in fact, this is generally untrue. The nerves that go to the nipple don't run along the surface of the breast, but rather come out of the rib cage and travel straight through the center of the breast to the nipple. The nerve trunk should not be in any greater danger during this procedure than with any other. As I mentioned in Chapter Four, it is my belief that the loss or gain in nipple sensation from breast implant surgery is likely caused by the position of the implant creating pressure on the nerve trunk. Some physicians suggest that this incision may reduce a patient's ability to breast-feed, but no definitive studies support this claim.

Another major advantage of the periareolar technique that cannot be dismissed is that it allows the surgeon to correct nipple asymmetry, or any other minor pre-existing position problems with the nipples, in the same surgery session. For example, if the nipples are too far to the outside, the surgeon will make the incision on the inside border of the nipple, take a small amount of skin from the breast along the line of the incision, and then pull the nipple across when it's time to close. Since breast augmentation will always increase any nipple asymmetry, and especially increase the problem if the nipples are too far to the outside, this is a very important benefit to the final look of your breasts.

FURTHER CONSIDERATIONS

TO SUMMARIZE ALL of the above information on breast augmentation surgery, you have three major decisions to make prior to your surgery. You will need to decide what type of implants the surgeon will use, how large they will be, and what surgical technique will be used to place them within your breasts. I generally recommend the round, saline-filled implants of a size that will look natural even if they are very large, placed in the submuscular position using a periareolar incision site. However, every case is different and every woman is different and in the end only you can make the final decisions on these options. The information presented in this chapter should help you have an informed discussion with your doctor, and together, hopefully, you will discover what is right for you. Though these are the major considerations, there are a few more things that you should know prior to your surgery.

As I mentioned earlier, it is no problem for most surgeons to make very pretty, nicely shaped breasts into larger, pretty, nicely shaped breasts. It is important in your consultation with your doctor that you discuss your goals and whether or not implant surgery alone will accomplish those goals. In many cases it will. In other cases, however, other sculpting techniques will be required. For example, extra fat, especially in and around the armpits, can frequently affect the shape of the breast and some simple liposuction to sculpt the shape of the breast can vastly improve the look of your breast augmentation. Sometimes a more complex solution is needed such as doing both an augmentation and a lift. Both liposuction and lifts are covered in Chapter Nine and Chapter Ten, and I recommend that you read them as well.

Another consideration that you should keep in mind is that the nipple is part of the skin of your breast and that any increase in the size of your breast will stretch the skin and therefore increase the size of the nipple. For many women this is not a concern. However, if you feel very strongly that you don't want larger nipples or that you would even like your nipples to be smaller, this will be an important factor to keep in mind. It is possible for your surgeon to correct this situation during a periareolar implant procedure by trimming the size of the nipple at the same time, but this will necessitate a scar that travels the entire edge of the nipple. Furthermore, this scar will potentially be more visible since, in reducing the size of the nipple, the color change, which is normally gradual between the nipple and skin surrounding it, will be more abrupt and clearly defined.

Another thing that you may have heard of and may have some curiosity about is the **"no touch technique."** This technique has generated some buzz over the last couple of years as a method for reducing the occurrence of noticeable capsular contracture. In the "no touch technique," the object is for the surgeon to never come in contact with the implant and even minimize any contact between the implant and the physician's surgical instruments—essentially getting the implant directly from it's package into the breast (usually with an antibiotic bath in between to protect against infection). Whether or not this procedure is actually effective in reducing capsular contracture is still unknown at this time, as no long-term studies have been completed on it. I have adopted the procedure in most cases since I can see no downside or risk associated with it.

WHAT WILL IT BE LIKE AFTER SURGERY?

ALL OF THE ABOVE involve decisions you must make before your surgery. Once you have made all of your decisions and you are ready to go ahead with your procedure you may be curious about what to expect afterwards.

As mentioned in Chapter Four, you should be prepared for a substantial amount of pain during the first day or two after surgery, especially with the submuscular procedure. Your doctor can prepare you for this eventuality by providing you with a prescription for pain medication. Your doctor may also provide you with a **pain pump**. This is a device that slowly releases an anesthetic directly into the muscle over a forty-eight-hour period. It is a more expensive option, but it is highly recommended because it is perfectly safe and extremely effective. You should also make your own preparations by organizing your life and your home prior to your surgery so that you will have time to recover without having to take care of things like shopping, cooking, or childcare. Please refer to "Your Pre- and Post-Surgery Checklist" in the back of this book for a complete list of things to consider.

The surgery will probably take about an hour. Your breasts will be tender and swollen, and you will have bandages and possibly tape over the area of incision. Your doctor will advise you in the proper care of the bandages based on how he has treated the area and also tell you when it is safe to bathe. Most of the time you will have to return after a few days to have some stitches removed but this is a generally simple and painless procudure, and most of the stitches are specially made to dissolve and absorb into your body to minimize scar appearance.

During the initial healing period, you will have to wear postoperative breast bands (large elastic bands around your chest to keep your implants in place); otherwise they have a tendency to rise toward your collarbone after surgery. You will need to wear the bands for two weeks. You will probably be able to resume light activity in two to four weeks and more vigorous exercise in six to eight weeks. You should not lift weights for at least six weeks. You should probably wait about five days before any air travel (and you should certainly not carry any heavy luggage for two weeks). Driving might be possible in about a week. If you're very careful, you can probably resume sexual relations in about a week as well. The amount of time for each of these is variable and depends on your surgery, how quickly you heal, how you feel, and what your doctor recommends.

To aid in healing and help prevent hard capsule formation, I have my patients massage their breasts for a minimum of five minutes, at least twice a day for the first six months after surgery. But that is a minimum. The more frequently you massage, the better for the healing process. In order to make sure that my patients manage to fit time into their day to do this I recommend that they to massage their breasts while in the bathroom or while stopped at a red light.

After several weeks, the swelling will subside and you'll start to see your final results. If you have followed all of the recommendations in this book you will almost certainly be very, very happy. The scar at the incision site will already be fairly subtle and it will continue to fade for up to six months or even a year. Most women who undergo breast augmentation are more pleased than they expected, and during the initial period of getting used to their new, curvier body, they have a great deal of fun in discovering how they look in different types of tops and dresses—frequently many items that they could not have worn previously.

Your doctor will tell you when follow-up visits are no longer necessary, and it might soon be easy to forget that you have implants at all. Of course, your breasts will not be protected against the normal stresses of aging, childbirth, or weight fluctuations any more than natural breasts and, as I have mentioned, your implants will eventually have to be replaced, but you will most likely be very happy for many years.

The Silicone Implant Controversy

Or How Trial Lawyers Created Mass Hysteria Based on Anecdotes and Deception

I T WAS MORE than a quarter century ago when the first woman filed a lawsuit against the manufacturer of her silicone breast implants for pain and suffering after her implants ruptured. She received $170,000. Twenty years ago, Ralph Nader's Washington-based Public Citizen Health Research Group issued warnings that silicone-filled implants caused cancer. In 1992, the FDA decided that silicone presented enough of a threat that it issued a ruling that women could no longer receive silicone gel implants except in cases of reconstruction, and only then as part of a large study group. By 1993, more than twelve thousand individuals, convinced of the danger, had filed lawsuits against Dow Corning, one of the largest American silicone implant manufacturers. A giant class-action suit settlement was finalized in March of 1994 against all silicone breast implant manufacturers. By 1995, an amazing 440,000 women had joined the class action, Dow Corning had declared bankruptcy, and other major pharmaceutical companies involved in the action—Baxter, Bristol-Myers, Squibb, and 3M—were all driven from the implant manufacturing business.

Yet, despite all of these lawsuits, billions of dollars paid out in settlements, the bankruptcy of a one of the largest pharmaceutical companies in the world, and hundreds of thousands of women complaining of diseases caused by their implants, the FDA is again allowing women to obtain silicone-filled implants for cosmetic breast augmentation. Why? Because after many studies on the nearly two million women with silicone breast implants in this country, in spite of all of the money paid out in settlements, the scientific community has found that there is absolutely no evidence that any of the problems that the hundreds of thousands of women have blamed on their implants were actually caused by their implants! In other words, the FDA has determined that the silicone implants are safe for use in cosmetic surgery.

This raises an enormous number of questions. Why would so many women claim that their implants made them sick if there wasn't something to it? Surely some might lie to make some money in a lawsuit—but just as surely not all *440,000 women!* If the implants are safe, why were billions of dollars paid out? Why did most of the large pharmaceutical companies stop manufacturing them? Why do most plastic surgeons, myself included, generally recommend against them? And just what is silicone anyway?

The best place to start is with that last question. Silicone is a polymer, a large, complex molecule made up of many smaller molecules. Imagine a train car as a molecule made up of many parts—wheels, windows, seats, etc. A polymer would be the entire train, made up of many train cars. In the case of silicone, the train car is a molecule made with the basic element, silicon. When these silicon-based molecules are strung together in long and complex chains, the result is a silicone. Many types of silicones are made by stringing together different lengths and different types of silicon-based molecules and adding other elements into the mix. Thus, silicone can be anything from a hard plastic to an industrial lubricant, to a soft gel resembling a "liquid rubber" that can be used in breast implants.

Silicon is the most common element on the planet. Beach sand is made from crystallized silica (silicon dioxide), and so is glass. Because of its incredible versatility, silicon is found in an amazing number of man-made products, from computer chips to common food stabilizers (most chocolate milk contains silica). Silicon naturally occurs inside the human body in fairly large quantities.

This is one reason why silicone is one of the best materials with which to make medical devices that are implanted into the body. The human body doesn't like anything foreign to be put inside it, but silicone polymers are among the best tolerated. Because there is a nearly infinite number of ways to make different silicones, medical scientists are always searching for new and better polymers of silicone that will be even better for use as medical implants. The silicone used in implants today is far better and more stable in the body than the silicone used in breast implants in the 1970s. That is just one of the reasons that the FDA is lifting its ban on silicone gel implants for cosmetic breast surgery.

The shell or bag of all breast implants is made from a silicone polymer, regardless of whether the implant is filled with saline or silicone gel. The material improvements to silicone are most evident in this material used to make the shell. The first implants made in the early sixties tended to rupture within the first few years. Today's implants are better in every way—they are far more durable, hold their shape better, and are better tolerated by the body.

Breast Surgery Fun Facts

WOMEN have injected various substances into their breasts to make them larger for more than a hundred years. Silicone was first used by Japanese prostitutes in the 1940's after World War II. But they were injecting the gel directly into the breast tissue, a very dangerous procedure. It wasn't until 1962 that Timmie Jean Lindsey became the first woman to receive silicone gel-filled breast implants.

WHY WERE SILICONE BREAST IMPLANTS BANNED, AND WAS THE BAN JUSTIFIED?

IN 1976, the FDA enacted the Medical Devices Amendment. The amendment required medical devices, such as implants, to be approved by the FDA for safety and effectiveness, just like prescription drugs. However, the Medical Devices Amendment had a grandfather clause that allowed devices that were already in common use to avoid FDA review unless their safety was called into question. Since silicone breast implants had already been in use for more than a decade, they were allowed to continue to be used without FDA approval. In fact, it wasn't until a decade later, in June 1988, that the FDA decided that the manufacturers of breast implants would be required to submit scientific studies to prove their safety.

The FDA gave the pharmaceutical companies three years to conduct their studies and compile data to show that silicone implants were safe. In July 1991, when the results were due, Dow Corning provided the FDA with the data from 329 studies. But after careful review, the FDA found that the studies were ultimately inconclusive. They could not prove that the silicone gel-filled implants were either safe or harmful. A year later, in

1992, still unsure whether or not silicone gel-filled implants were inherently dangerous, the FDA banned the use of the implants for cosmetic surgery. For the next two decades the only women who could receive silicone-filled implants in the United States were those undergoing reconstructive surgery, and then only as part of a scientific study.

During the course of the past twenty years, while the ban on silicone implants for cosmetic surgery has been in effect, billions of dollars in settlements have been paid out to thousands upon thousands of women who claimed that their silicone breast implants caused all sorts of diseases, from cancer to rheumatoid arthritis to lupus. But did the implants cause these diseases? Within the limits of scientific evidence gathered for nearly a half a century since the first implant procedure, the answer appears to be no.

Imagine for a moment that you have gone to a restaurant for lunch with a few of your friends. Later that afternoon you become nauseous and by evening you are feverish and vomiting. If you are like most people you will assume that something that you ate at that restaurant made you sick. In all likelihood, you'll never go back to that place and you'll tell your friends to avoid it as well, assuming that the place gave you food poisoning.

But the truth is, it may have been something you ate at breakfast or even something from dinner the night before that was tainted with a virus that didn't amplify enough in your body to make you sick until the following day. In fact, it's just as likely that you came in contact with somebody with a virus, maybe shook his or her hand or accepted some money or something else that the person touched, and contracted the virus in this way. In other words, even though you will probably blame the restaurant for making you sick, it is very likely that you got sick someplace else. But it's human nature to see the cause and effect in things. It's nearly impossible to not suspect the restaurant if you became sick right after eating there.

The same thing seems to have occurred with silicone breast implants. When somebody gets a horrible, life-wrecking disease like cancer, rheumatoid arthritis, or lupus, she naturally asks why. Many question their awful luck; they'll even ask God why this terrible punishment has been forced upon them.

Now imagine that you are a woman who has been healthy her whole life, and shortly after receiving silicone gel-filled implants you are diagnosed with a dreaded disease like lupus. No doctor knows why some people get lupus and others don't. It is a very mysterious disease whose cause is unknown. But you were perfectly healthy before you got those silicone implants. How could you not draw a line of cause and effect between the chemicals in those implants and the sudden occurrence of lupus? Likewise, if you had heard of someone's friend who two years after receiving her implants was suddenly diagnosed with cancer, it might very well give you some doubts about getting implants yourself.

For thousands of women, this is exactly what happened. So how can it be that scientists say that it is *not* the implants that caused the diseases? This illusion was created by the incredibly large number of women who received silicone gel-filled implants—over 1.5 million in the United States alone. That's a number that is difficult for most people to understand. In a group of 1.5 million women with silicone implants, thousands became ill in the years following their surgery. But in a group of 1.5 million women who did not have any surgery, an almost *exactly identical number became sick* with the same types of diseases. In other words, there is no connection between having implant surgery and getting one of these terrible diseases. Patients with silicone implants did not have a higher risk for any of the diseases described in the class-action lawsuit. The numbers don't lie. A certain number of women will get sick in a group of millions—with or without implants. In fact, the percentage of women with breast cancer was substantially lower in the group with implants—though there is no evidence that implants have any role in preventing cancer!

SO DOES THIS MEAN THAT SILICONE GEL IMPLANTS ARE SAFE?

LITERALLY THOUSANDS OF STUDIES have been performed on the safety of implants. Some have examined the chemicals used in the implant shells and fillings, some have reviewed surgical complications, others have explored the link between implants and connective tissue diseases. Still others have covered diverse subjects like the effects of mammography radiation on breast implants and the effect of implants on breast milk. How did the FDA sift through all of this information to reach its conclusions?

In 1997, the United States House of Representatives told the Department of Health and Human Services to sort out the safety issues of silicone breast implants. The Institute of Medicine (IOM) was given the mission of assembling a panel of top scientists from various medical fields, from immunology to neurology to plastic surgery and many others, to sort through all of the studies available, devise some of their own if necessary, and report back on their findings. It was on the basis of these findings that the FDA has reapproved the use of silicone implants.

I'll start with the good news about what the panel found: Silicone breast implants do not cause cancer, or connective tissue disorders, or autoimmune diseases like rheumatoid arthritis or lupus. There was great consistency among all of the studies reviewed on this subject. Furthermore, there have been suggestions (primarily from lawyers, not doctors) that silicone breast implants may cause some new class of diseases, silicone specific diseases that had been previously unclassified. The studies showed absolutely no evidence for the existence of any of these diseases.

The panel also found that the breast milk of women who had received silicone breast implants was perfectly safe for infants. As I mentioned in Chapter Six, there may be complications with breast-feeding for women who have had cosmetic breast surgery unrelated to implants, but if a woman is able to breast-feed after her surgery, there is no reason to believe that there are any health concerns for the baby. Many studies have shown that breast milk is the best food for babies. Women with silicone breast implants are no exception to this rule. While slightly elevated levels of silicon have been found in the breast milk of these women, it is still significantly *lower* than the amount of silicon found in cows' milk or commercially available baby formula.

Furthermore, silicone implants can't harm a developing fetus. There had been some worry that silicon from the implant could cross from the mother's bloodstream into the placenta. In fact, there is no increased level of silicon in the blood of women with silicone implants. More importantly, there is no evidence of an increase in the number of birth defects for women with silicone implants compared to women without implants.

Another concern addressed by the panel was the worry that the radiation from mammography or other X-ray procedures might somehow affect the silicone used in the implants—either the shell or the gel inside. There have been some published reports that radiation might weaken the implants or that the implants might interfere with radiation therapy. All of these fears were found to be baseless. In fact, radiation has been found to have no effect on implants and vice versa, implants have been found to have no affect on radiation therapy. However, there is some speculation that radiation therapy might cause an increase in the occurrence of capsular contracture (See Chapter Four, "Risks and Rewards" and Chapter Seven, "Breast Enlargement" for a complete explanation of capsular contracture and its role in assessing the risks of breast augmentation surgery.). So the jury is still out and more research must be done in this area. In the interim, it is something to consider for women thinking about silicone implants.

Finally, the results of the panel suggest that, chemically, silicone is generally safe. In the doses reasonably expected to be found in women with silicone implants, silicone does not appear to present any kind of health threat. Silicone is found in a wide variety of products and has been in common use for many decades. Some level of silicon is found in all humans without any health consequences. Even in women whose silicone implants have ruptured, exposure to silicon seems to be limited to the areas of the breast immediately surrounding the implant.

All of this is indeed good news. Based on these findings, the FDA is again going to allow women to receive silicone-filled implants. However, not all the news was good, and there are still some concerns related to silicone-filled implants and breast implants in general. I've addressed most of these concerns in Chapter Four and Chapter Seven, but I'll briefly repeat them here with specific reference to the findings of the IOM Committee. The most important fact regarding the silicone controversy and the dangers of silicone implants is that there is no evidence that silicone causes any kind of illness to the body as a whole. All of the dangers associated with silicone implants are dangers that are local to the area immediately surrounding the implant itself and the surgical site and areas affected by the surgery.

The biggest danger addressed by the panel is that breast implants do not last forever. While this is not a problem specifically associated with silicone, silicon, or silicone gel-filled implants, it is nevertheless a real risk to women with implants of any variety. Implants will eventually rupture. In the case of silicone implants, rupturing frequently goes undetected because the silicone remains within the capsule formed by the body. It is unclear if a rupture of this nature that goes unnoticed could result in some long-term risks or local complications in the breast. In cases where the rupture is detected (as in the deflation of a saline implant), surgery will be required to replace the implant. While this surgery is much simpler and less painful than the initial implant surgery, there are always risks associated with surgery. Another piece of good news for women now considering breast implants is that the implants used today are far better than those used in years gone by, and they can be expected to last much longer. However, no implant is permanent, and the risk of an implant failing increases over time.

Additionally, the rupture of a silicone implant sometimes results in the silicone gel escaping into other tissue near the breast where it becomes encapsulated by the body. This can result in an unwanted lump in other areas of the chest, the armpit, or even in the arm itself. This could require surgical correction, removal of the implant and capsule and escaped silicone, and probably the insertion of a new implant. Just like your original surgery, this entails risks, possibly hematoma and infection.

Conversely, because the rupture of a silicone implant frequently goes undetected, the IOM panel left an open question as to whether some test or protocol should be devised to determine when or if an implant has ruptured. The fact that ruptures are not always detected, combined with the fact that a wide variety of different silicone materials have been used for implant shells has made it almost impossible for the panel to determine what the actual chances are that a new implant will rupture during any given period of time. Some investigations of the latest types of implants (sometimes referred to as third generation implants) have seen no evidence of any ruptures at all, but of course these implants are newer and there are no long-term studies of them as yet. Other studies have shown more frequent rupturing and deflation than expected. As a general rule, most women with breast implants will outlive their implants, whether filled with saline or silicone gel.

Perhaps the largest real problem with silicone-filled implants as opposed to saline is the increased incidence of severe capsular contracture. As discussed in Chapter Four, all women with implants experience some degree of capsular contracture. For most women, the amount of contracture that occurs is acceptable and not very noticeable. In other women, who experience a higher degree of capsular contracture, the results can be very bad, both in the appearance and the feel of the breast, and can even result in pain. This will more than likely require additional surgery to correct.

One of the most important points to make here is that doctors and scientists don't know what causes severe capsular contracture or why some women develop more severe contracture than others. Because of this ongoing uncertainty and because of the many variables involved, from the composition of the implant shell to the placement of the implant within the breast, to the different surgical procedures involved, there is still no certainty as to whether silicone gel implants do indeed cause an increase in capsular contracture and, if so, just how much of a greater risk exists. However, it does appear that silicone gel-filled implants do have a higher incidence of developing a thicker capsule. This is the main reason that most surgeons do not recommend them for their patients.

All of this uncertainty just tends to feed the ongoing controversy surrounding silicone gel implants. Furthermore, much more than science is involved in this controversy. Lawyers, with very definitive, non-scientific goals are involved, as are feminists, psychologists, and sociologists—all of whom have their own motivations and political concerns regarding women taking risks to change their appearance. This is no simple issue, and I can't pretend to have all of the answers.

From a scientific point of view, while there are some definitive conclusions to the silicone implant controversy, these conclusions do not change the moral and psychological issues surrounding the subject. For many women these scientific conclusions are very unsatisfying because it leaves them without an explanation for their illnesses. The sad truth is that the world is filled with events, some tragic, that science simply can't yet explain. It is tempting to blame whatever (or whomever) is at hand. Some women with breast implants are in fact very ill, but there is simply no evidence that their implants are the reason that they are sick.

Breast Reduction
Relieve the Burden

O F THE VARIOUS cosmetic procedures available for
the breast, breast reduction is the only one that is frequently
deemed a medical necessity and thus frequently covered by
insurance. While some women elect to have their breasts
reduced in size for purely aesthetic considerations, it is more
common that women seeking breast reductions are doing so
for persuasive medical or social reasons. Women with
extremely large breasts—breasts that are simply too big for
their frame and proportions—frequently experience chronic
and onerous back and neck pain. Sometimes the weight of
their breasts can also lead to painful shoulder grooving from
bra straps and severe, chronic skin rashes. Excessively large
breasts can prevent a woman from participating in many enjoyable and healthful physical activities. Additionally, women with

excessively large breasts may face psychosocial pressures that can lead to very real psychological and emotional injury. There are a variety of surgical solutions to reducing the volume of breast tissue. Many of them are also associated with a breast lift to compensate for the reduction in tissue and for the sagging that occurs from the breasts' excessive volume. I suggest you read both this chapter and the following chapter if you're interested in reducing the size of your breasts.

DETERMINING THE PROCEDURE
THAT'S BEST FOR YOU

IN VERY FEW cases, a reduction can be accomplished with some simple liposuction sculpting. The success of this technique depends on a couple of factors. One has to do with the percentage of fat in the breasts as opposed to gland tissue. Every woman is different in this case, but if your breasts are composed of mostly gland tissue with very little fat, liposuction would be ruled out as a means of reduction. Liposuction, when used successfully, is an excellent option because it is minimally invasive, which translates to lower risks, less discomfort, a shorter recovery, and minimum scarring.

If your breasts are large but not yet sagging, and, specifically, if your nipples are in a normal position, then you might be a good candidate for reduction by liposuction. Most women who require a reduction have some degree of breast ptosis, or sagging. Usually the amount of ptosis is defined in terms of the diagonal distance, in centimeters, from the notch at the base of the neck where the collar bones come together. These measurements are expressed in ranges and are only generalizations, since a very tall woman would anticipate a generally larger distance than a very petite woman, but they are a good rule of thumb.

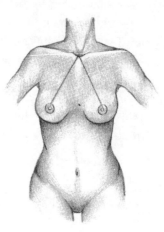

Measurements from the sternal notch to the nipple will help to assess your degree of ptosis (sagging) and the procedures available to you.

If your nipples are more than twenty-one centimeters from the notch in the breastbone you will most likely require surgery beyond what can be achieved with liposuction. Since tissue other than fat will need to be removed, an incision must be made and, as in breast enlargement, the surgeon will attempt to place the scar in an area where it is least noticeable.

THE MCKISSOCK TECHNIQUE

UNTIL RECENTLY, the method of choice was to remove the skin around the nipple in a "keyhole" pattern. The volume of unwanted tissue is removed and the remaining tissue is pulled together inside the breast. The nipple, still attached to the tissue, nerves, and blood supply beneath it, is simply drawn upward to the top of the incision area and then the skin from the sides is pulled and stitched together beneath the breast. Matching the sides is not so very different from stitching the flat pieces from a sewing pattern to create a desired three-dimensional shape. This keyhole pattern is sometimes referred to as either the **McKissock technique** or the **Wise pattern**. The resulting scar resembles an anchor, or some say an inverted T, drawn beneath the nipple.

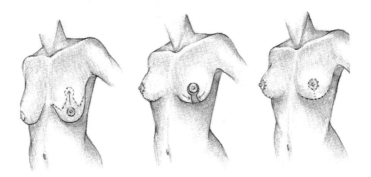

The Wise pattern breast reduction procedure removes skin and breast tissue. The nipple is lifted to the desired position, leaving an anchor-shaped scar. This technique leaves a boxy-shaped breast that tends to bottom-out (breast tissue sags below the nipple).

While in some cases the McKissock technique is still preferred, it does have some shortcomings. First is, obviously, the anchor-shaped scar. Not only are there additional scars, but because the skin at the bottom of the breast—the inframammary fold—is thicker than the rest of the breast skin, it tends to make a thicker, more visually obvious scar, sometimes developing an hypertrophic or **keloid scar**. Also, since the scar is directly underneath the underwire of the patient's bra it is also extremely uncomfortable. For women seriously in need of a large reduction in breast volume this will probably seem like a small price to pay, but it is a larger scar than most women, and most surgeons, would prefer.

Another drawback to the McKissock technique is that some women feel that the resulting shape of the breast is somewhat "boxy." Since breast shape is such a subjective matter, it is always important to see your surgeon's before-and-after patient photographs to determine whether you like his or her work. The McKissock technique is also sometimes associated with the breast "bottoming-out" after surgery. That is, the tissue of the breast drops downward and stretches the skin at the bottom of the breast, causing the nipple to point upwards. This causes an associated loss in **breast projection** (the medical term for how far your breasts protrude).

CIRCUMAREOLAR INCISION

AS A RESULT of dissatisfaction among patients and surgeons, some new techniques have been pioneered that yield cosmetically better results. The technique that leaves the most well-hidden scar is the **circumareolar incision** around the nipple. This is an excellent option for women seeking a breast reduction whose nipples are located between twenty-one and twenty-five centimeters from the collarbone. The surgeon makes his opening in an oval shape that extends above the nipple. The unwanted volume of breast tissue is removed and then the nipple, still attached to the tissue below, is lifted to the top of the incision, and the skin is drawn together around it in the same manner as cinching the top of a purse together with a drawstring. This is actually referred to by surgeons as the **purse-string stitching technique**.

When the top of a purse is pulled together with a drawstring, the opening puckers together. Nobody wants the skin around their nipple to pucker together, so plastic surgeons have devised special stitching techniques that help the skin to

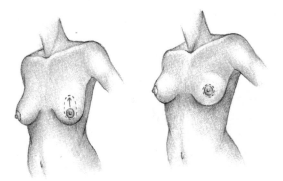

The Goës technique for a breast reduction or lift is useful for smaller breasts and has a scar that only encircles the areola. This technique yields a moderately projecting breast.

lay flat giving a very natural look to women who have had this procedure. In some cases, further support can be given to the remaining tissue that has been drawn together within the breast by placing a fine mesh that, over time, absorbs into the body. This circumareolar technique with a mesh support is sometimes referred to as the **Goës technique** for Dr. Joao Sampaio Goës, the Brazilian surgeon who pioneered it, and it yields excellent results. The ability to elevate the nipple and redistribute the breast tissue is excellent, however projection of the breast tissue is only fair.

The limitation is that for women whose nipples are below the twenty-five centimeter mark, the size of the circular piece of skin that is removed from around the nipple increases until it becomes impossible to cinch the skin together without some puckering around the nipple. Every case is different, and women with very youthful and elastic skin may be able to go a bit larger, but generally for women whose nipples are below twenty-five centimeters, another technique must be used.

VERTICAL SCAR BREAST REDUCTION

FOR THE ABOVE reasons, women seeking a reduction whose nipples are between twenty-five and thirty-three centimeters beneath the notch in the breastbone will usually opt for a **vertical scar breast reduction**, sometimes referred to as the **Lejour technique** for Madeleine Lejour, the French surgeon who pioneered it. The advantages to this procedure are a smaller scar and less boxy breast shape than the McKissock technique. The surgeon removes the smallest amount of skin possible, but enough to move the nipple to a more desirable position. This skin removal pattern typically appears like a dome situated on top of a vertically oriented oval. The desired volume of tissue is then removed in a wedge at the bottom of the breast and the remaining tissue is brought together, folded inward, and stitched together. Then the nipple is placed in the circle above and the sides of the skin are brought together.

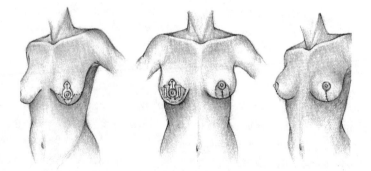

The vertical reduction mammoplasty, or the Lejour technique, is one version of the "lollipop" scar breast reduction. This technique creates a round-shaped breast with excellent projection.

When put together at the end of surgery, the scar is often called a "lollipop" scar because of its lollipop-like shape. Most patients find that this unobtrusive vertical scar that descends from the nipple to the base of the breast acceptable. The resulting breast usually has a beautiful shape and the scar, over time, will usually fade quite dramatically when compared to the anchor-shaped scar associated with the McKissock technique.

The Lejour technique creates a breast that is full at the top and has more forward projection—a shape that most patients prefer. You can get a sense of this fullness at the top and forward projection on your own breast by taking your hand and cupping your breast from the bottom and squeezing the skin together, forcing the tissue up and outward. This will show the approximate shape of the breast after the surgery, but it obviously will not show the new, higher position of the nipple.

Variations of this technique have become commonplace in the recent past, which is a testimonial to the importance of this new procedure. A common variation, known as the **Hall-Findlay technique**, uses the same skin incision but leaves the nipple attached to the inner half of the breast tissue, reducing the breast by removing tissue from the outer half of the breast. This technique has several benefits, including shorter operating time and a better blood supply to the nipple. It is also useful when you have incisions on your breasts from breast biopsies (a fairly frequent occurrence). The major limitation is that the projection is not as great as with the Lejour technique and the scar may take longer to settle to its final look.

Be advised: Vertical scar techniques are more difficult to learn and have a steep learning curve. Be certain that if this is what your doctor suggests for you, that he or she has had a lot of experience with the technique and refer to Chapter Five, to "Choosing a Surgeon," for more on the physician selection process.

THE FREE-NIPPLE PROCEDURE

UNFORTUNATELY, THOUGH THE vertical scar breast reduction procedure is a good option, not every woman is a good candidate for it. When the breast volume is too great and the nipple is more than thirty-three centimeters from the top of the chest, it is impossible to remove enough tissue using only the lollipop scar and the surgeon will be forced to resort to a technique, like the McKissock technique, that creates an anchor-shaped scar. In extreme cases, a free-nipple procedure might be necessary. In this case, so much tissue needs to be removed from the breast and the nipple is so far below where it will ultimately be placed that the surgeon is not able to leave the nipple attached to the tissue beneath it, and it must be actually removed and then reattached in its new position. For women who require this type of surgery, the resulting anchor-shaped scar (or even the additional risk of the free-nipple procedure) is usually well worthwhile for the relief that they experience and the general improvement in their lives resulting from this surgery.

WHAT TO EXPECT

UNLESS YOU ARE a candidate for a reduction using only liposuction, a breast reduction is usually considered a more serious surgical procedure than a simple augmentation with an implant and will usually require an overnight stay in the hospital. However, with the restrictions now being placed on hospitals by insurance companies, patients receiving reductions are quite often discharged the same day as surgery in spite of the doctor's wishes or good judgment. As with an augmentation, it is very important that you prepare your body for the surgery by getting good sleep and nutrition in the week prior to your procedure. If you are a smoker, quit. If you cannot quit, you should at least be prepared not to smoke for at least three weeks prior to and following your surgery. Women taking any kind of immunosuppressive medications, have difficulty with healing, or have any current infections should delay or cancel their surgery until these matters can be resolved. And finally, as with a breast augmentation, it is important to arrange your life prior to your surgery so that you will have time to properly recover without the responsibilities of childcare, work, or meal preparation. Please see "Your Pre- and Post-Surgery Checklist" at the back of this book for a list o things to keep in mind.

After your surgery, your surgeon will prescribe medication to help you deal comfortably with soreness and swelling. Within the first week you will experience a certain amount of discomfort, and you should expect swelling and bruising in the area. It will take several weeks before you can stop wearing a special support bra and for normal sensation to return to your nipples, and for you to return to most normal activities and exercise. In a few months' time, your breasts will settle into their new shape. Your scars will begin to fade and, if you had been suffering from chronic back and neck pain, you will finally experience relief!

In addition to back and neck pain, many women with very large breasts are simply unable to exercise, and as a result they may gain weight and tire easily. After breast reduction surgery, many of these patients successfully lose weight and establish healthful exercise regiments that previously they couldn't have imagined.

Breast reduction usually makes a very dramatic difference in a woman's life and in her self-image. It may take some time to get used to your form, but overwhelmingly, women who have had breast reduction surgery are extremely satisfied with the results and the new doors that it opens.

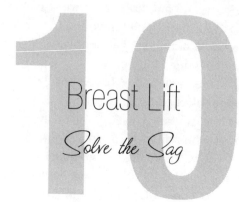

Breast Lift
Solve the Sag

THE TECHNIQUES USED for a breast lift are very similar to those used for a reduction. As with the reduction, there is a lifting of the internal tissue and raising of the nipple, but obviously with the breast lift there is little or no reduction of breast volume. In fact, breast lifts are often combined with augmentation to both lift and fill sagging breasts. This technique is at the forefront of new techniques in breast surgery, so it is extremely important to study this chapter prior to seeing your surgeon. This chapter will discuss breast lifts with the various scar techniques as well as lifts with augmentation

The original technique used for a breast lift, sometimes called the **Goulian mastopexy**, involved taking the skin around the nipple in the same McKissock technique or Wise pattern that is used in a breast reduction, and then simply drawing the skin together below the nipple, without removing or sculpting any of the internal breast tissue. The idea was to use the tightened skin to form a "skin bra." The problem with this technique is that since nothing is done to lift the tissue inside the breast and since none of the tissue is removed, as in the reduction technique, it does not take very long for the skin to stretch back into its original shape—now accented with an anchor-shaped scar.

The choice of surgical technique for a breast lift will depend to some degree on the amount of ptosis or sagging that must be corrected. Generally, we divide the degree of ptosis into four types:

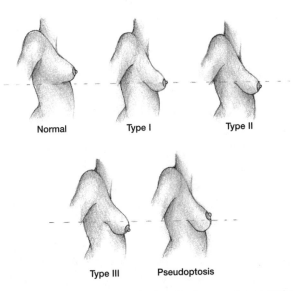

Breast ptosis classifications: Type I is described as sagging when the nipple areolar complex (NAC) is at the level of the inframammary fold; Type II is when the NAC is below this line; Type III is when the NAC points toward the floor; Pseudoptosis is when the breast tissue sags below the inframammary fold, but the NAC remains above the fold.

In a well-shaped breast, the nipple usually sits above the level of the inframammary fold. (As you may recall from earlier chapters, the inframammary fold is where the underside of the breast attaches to the chest). Type I ptosis refers to a breast where the nipple has descended to approximately the same level as the inframammary fold. When the nipple has fallen below the fold, it is called type II ptosis. Type III ptosis is when the nipple is not only below the fold, but actually points downward. The fourth form of ptosis is more unusual and is called **pseudoptosis**.

A breast with pseudoptosis has the nipple in correct position above the inframammary fold, but the tissue beneath the nipple has dropped out beneath it. Examples of the different types of ptosis can be seen in figure eighteen on page 109.

For type I ptosis and in some cases of type II ptosis, the circumareolar Goës procedure is the preferred technique. With this Brazilian procedure, as discussed in the previous chapter on breast reduction, the surgeon enters through an incision around the nipple to minimize scarring. An oval of skin is removed, allowing the surgeon to raise the nipple, and the tissue within the breast is physically raised, sculpted, and anchored into position by suturing it to the chest wall. Usually an absorbable mesh is used to further stabilize the tissue. Then the skin is brought together around the nipple in a purse-string fashion. This procedure has been shown to provide a very soft, natural-looking breast with much more durable results than the old Goulian mastopexy. As I have previously mentioned, this technique only creates moderate breast projection.

For women with type III ptosis, the Lejour technique (lollipop scar), is preferred. If you are a woman who has type II ptosis but you desire the greater projection and fullness that are achieved with the Lejour technique, you may be willing to live with the small additional scar to achieve this result. As in the reduction procedure, this technique yields a lollipop scar that fades over time, but will never completely disappear. The surgeon removes the skin in a circle above the nipple (where the nipple will ultimately be placed) and in a wedge beneath. The tissue of the breast is sculpted, sutured to the chest wall above, and brought together from below. A mesh may be placed within the breast to give greater support—much like an internal bra. Then the nipple, still attached to the tissue below, is raised to its new position and the skin is brought together below and stitched in place. The Lejour procedure gives so much projection that many women who have this procedure appear to have much larger breasts afterwards. In fact, many women who believe that they need an augmentation with an implant along with a breast lift find that because they actually had enough breast volume (but in the wrong place), the shape achieved with the Lejour-style lift alone is satisfactory and they opt not to have the implant.

BREAST LIFTS WITH IMPLANTS

DO IMPLANTS HAVE a role in breast lift procedures? Yes. For some women with minimal ptosis and small breasts, an implant may be used in place of a breast lift. The idea is to "fill out" the breast sufficiently to negate the need for the additional scars and surgery required by a breast lift. While this sounds very reasonable, it is in fact very unusual that this technique produces satisfactory results. Even with a circumareolar incision, which allows the surgeon to raise the nipple, the sagging tissue and skin of the breast usually falls below the implant. One of my patients described this as the "rock-in-the-sock" look. In order to fill out the extra skin and tissue properly, the implant will usually have to be far larger than most women want when they first consider this procedure.

The Difference Implants Can Make

I MET a beautiful, statuesque woman at a party once who, after finding out what I did for a living, told me all about her procedure. She had small sagging breasts that she had felt horrible about, but she was absolutely terrified by the prospect of cutting around or having any scars even near her nipples or breasts. She consulted with several surgeons and finally decided that the only possibility for her to lift her sagging breasts was to get implants through an axillary (underarm) incision. Though her breasts were quite small, the only way to properly fill them out was to use a very large implant, taking her from an A-cup all the way to a D-cup. In this woman's case, the results were good because she also happens to be 5'11" with a broad-shouldered, athletic frame. Since at first she had never intended to have a breast augmentation, it took some time for her to get used to her new proportions, which were much larger than she had ever anticipated. But, she confided to me, she absolutely loved her new body. Clearly not every woman would have felt the same way. As always with cosmetic breast surgery, it is a very personal decision.

Breast lifts combined with implants can be performed in many different ways with a diverse range of outcomes. Many surgeons feel that these procedures should be staged in two operations. At the first stage, an augmentation is performed. In the post-operative period patients are subject to all the risks of the augmentation procedure, but are still faced with the problem of sagging breasts, only they are bigger! In the second stage, the lift is performed, with all the risks of the first operation, only with the added cost in time and money.

Other surgeons believe that an augmentation with a skin excision around the areola is an adequate version of the combined augmentation-lift procedure. This technique involves

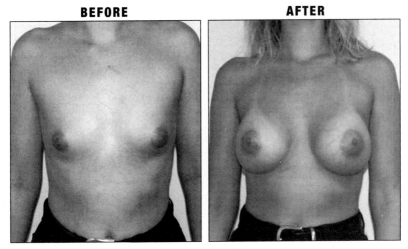

BEFORE   **AFTER**

Age: 25 | Height: 5'10"

425 cc round, smooth saline implants inserted using a periareolar incision. Although these are relatively large implants, the patient's height, chest wall dimensions, and pre-existing amount of breast tissue all contribute to the final breast size.

BEFORE   **AFTER**

Age: 23 | Height: 5'7"

350 cc round, smooth saline implants inserted using a periareolar incision. Outward pointing nipples were corrected using a crescent-shaped excision on the inner aspect of the areola. This technique corrects nipple asymmetry but leaves a more visible scar.

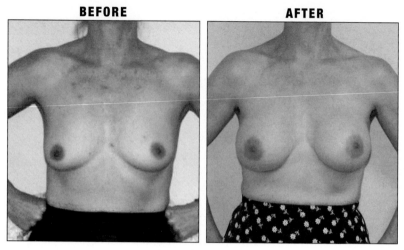

Age: 48 | Height: 5'7"

350 cc round, smooth saline implants inserted using a periareolar incision. A nice pre-surgical breast shape will yield a nice post-surgical breast shape.

BEFORE   **AFTER**

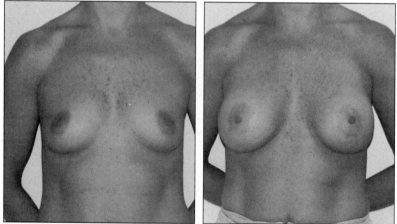

Age: 34 | Height: 5'4"

325 cc round, smooth saline implants inserted using a periareolar incision. The patient was looking for a moderate improvement without the typical "implant look."

Breast Enlargements

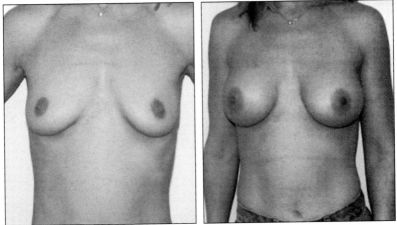

Age: 32 | Height: 5'7"

350 cc round, smooth saline implants inserted using a periareolar incision. In the before picture, note the moderate breast ptosis (sagging), caused by pregnancy and breast-feeding. In the after picture, the breasts look great, but still have the ptosis. In order to completely remove the breast ptosis, excessively large implants or a lift combined with an augmentation would be required.

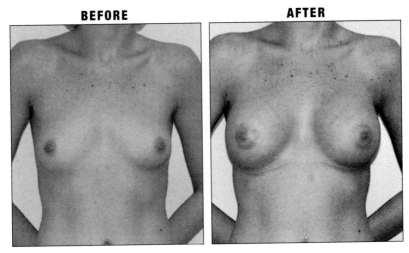

Age: 24 | Height: 5'4"

300 cc round, smooth saline implants inserted using a periareolar incision. The patient was looking for a moderate, natural-looking change. Not all implants have to be over-done!

BEFORE **AFTER**

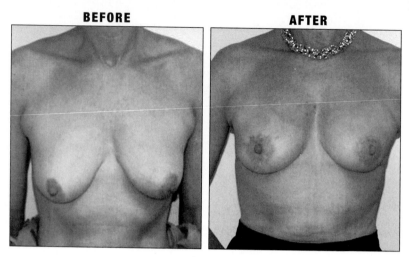

Age: 57 | Height: 5'6"

Lift performed using the Goës technique. The patient had type II ptosis. Note the moderate improvement in projection despite nice cleavage.

BEFORE **AFTER**

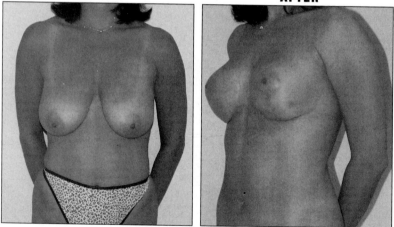

Age: 36 | Height: 5'6"

Lift performed using the Lejour vertical reduction technique with liposuction of the armpit area. The patient had type II ptosis and large pendulous breasts. The Lejour technique creates excellent projection compared to the Goës technique.

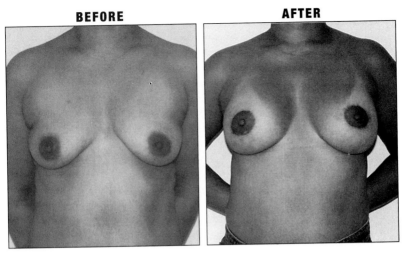

Age: 47 | Height: 5'4"

Lift performed using my own teardrop augmentation mastopexy. The upper poles of the breasts were narrowed and the lower poles were widened. Fat was removed from the armpit, which allowed for a moderate, natural-looking augmentation.

BEFORE **AFTER**

Age: 38 | Height: 5'2"

This patient, with severely sagging breasts after breastfeeding and giving birth to three babies, desired a modest enlargement with minimal scarring. My own teardrop augmentation mastopexy lifted and filled the upper poles of her breasts, creating a natural-looking enhancement.

Breast Lifts with Enlargements

BEFORE   **AFTER**

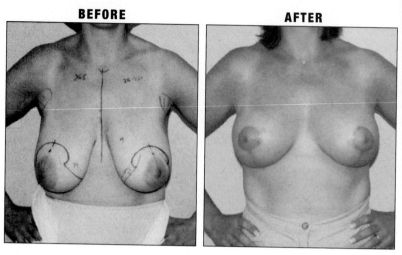

Age: 36 | Height: 5'4"

The patient had type II ptosis and pendulous breasts. The Lejour vertical reduction technique made them rounder and created excellent projection.

BEFORE   **AFTER**

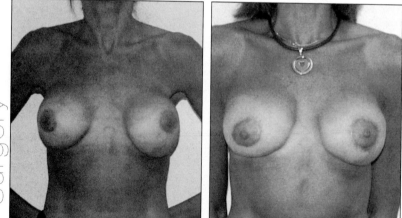

Age: 48 | Height: 5'1"

The patient had two previous breast augmentation attempts. The implants were replaced and moved from the subglandular position to the submuscular position. Scar tissue was removed, and the breasts' positions were corrected. The nipples were moved medially and the inframammary fold was elevated.

BEFORE **AFTER**

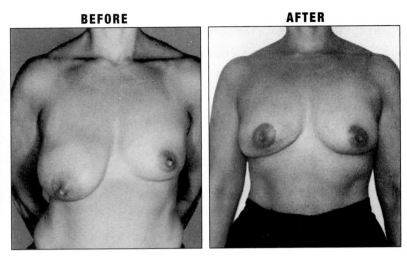

Age: 44 | Height: 5'3"

The patient's right breast was corrected using the Goës reduction technique. No surgery was performed on the left breast. Note the minimal scarring and that the areola on the surgically corrected side now matches the untouched side.

BEFORE **AFTER**

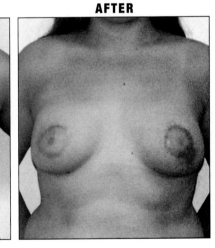

Age: 20 | Height: 5'5"

The patient, a smoker, had asymmetric, tubular breasts. Both breasts were enlarged using a circumareolar incision and breast implants of different sizes. Because the tubular breast has a narrow base, the breast mound was also widened. Note the scarring on the patient's left breast, a result of the smoking and its effect on blood supply and wound healing.

BEFORE   AFTER

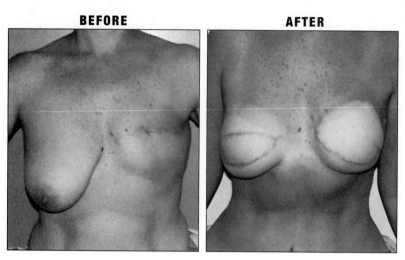

Age: 37 | Height: 5'4"

The patient had a mastectomy of her left breast and radiation, and needed a mastectomy of her right breast. Both breasts were reconstructed with TRAM flaps.

BEFORE   AFTER

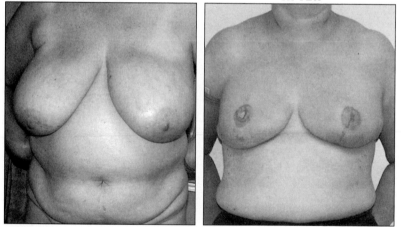

Age: 48 | Height: 5'9"

The patient's cancerous right breast was reconstructed by inserting tissue from the *latissimus dorsi* muscle, which runs down from the shoulder blade area of the back. An implant was placed under the muscle to enhance breast size. The left breast was reduced and a nipple-areola complex was created on the right breast by taking excess areola tissue from the left side.

removing as much skin as is necessary to lift the nipple to its desired new position and to reshape the sagging breast tissue. Augmentation-lift techniques using skin excision alone will give inconsistent results that may result in scarring, asymmetrical areolas, and generally poorly shaped breasts. With these warnings, perhaps it is more important to find the right doctor for breast lifts than for any other breast procedure.

For most women seeking a breast lift and augmentation, the techniques I've just mentioned rarely yield satisfactory results. However, implants can still be used very effectively in conjunction with breast lifts to yield very beautiful results. For example, a technique that I pioneered, called **teardrop augmentation mastopexy**, combines a modified Goës technique with a round saline implant placed beneath the chest muscle. I began using this technique in 1998, and recently presented my results to the

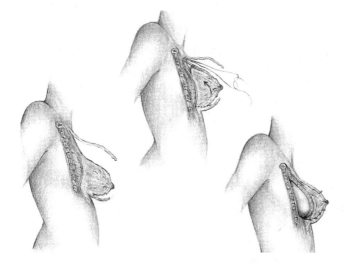

The teardrop augmentation mastopexy is a technique I created to correct sagging breasts that need a small increase in volume. The breast tissue is pulled above the implant, thereby filling out the upper chest, eliminating the pectoral shelf deformity. The scar only encircles the NAC.

International Society of Plastic Surgeons (Sydney, Australia) and The American Aesthetic Society (Boston, Massachusetts).

Because the tissue is sculpted both above and below the implant, the combination of the implant and breast tissue creates a teardrop-shaped breast. This technique creates a natural shape with excellent projection. Additionally, in patients with ptosis, the upper part of the chest is typically hollow. By reshaping the breast tissue, the hollowness is eliminated and a natural cleavage is formed. The lifting procedure eliminates the necessity for a large implant to fill the hollow sac, thus the volume of the implant can be precisely controlled to give the patient exactly the size that she wants. The end result is a very beautiful breast with a very natural yet dramatic "teardrop" silhouette.

Whether you are a better candidate for a lift alone or a lift with an implant is something that you can determine with your surgeon. Together you can discuss the situation and decide if your current breast volume, properly reproportioned and lifted, is sufficient.

LIPOSUCTION

LIPOSUCTION MAY ALSO play a role in a breast lift, even for women who are not initially interested in a reduction in volume. By decreasing the fat content of the breast a more firm and shapely breast can be created. The lower the fat content in the breasts, the less vulnerable they will be to fluctuations in body weight in the future. Women who desire a lift might also have small folds of excess fat in the armpit area that can form small rolls of skin when wearing a bra or swimsuit. Removing this extra fat with liposuction during the lift procedure allows a much more pleasing result.

PREPARATION AND WHAT TO EXPECT

THE PATIENT PREPARATIONS for the weeks leading up to the surgery and the duration of recovery are the same as for women seeking breast reductions, so look at Chapter Nine even if you are planning a lift or a lift and augmentation. Also refer to "Your Pre- and Post-Surgery Checklist" at the back of this book. At a minimum, you must stop smoking, eat and sleep well, and organize your life to allow yourself a stress-free period of healing following your surgery.

As always, you must have a realistic view of what cosmetic breast surgery can and can't offer you. Examine the photographs in the before-and-after section of this book to get a good idea of the type of results that are possible and what kind of scars you might expect. Different breast shapes will get different final results. It is your surgeon's job to show you portfolio photographs of patients with issues similar to yours.

Correcting Mismatched Breasts

You Are Not Alone

ASYMMETRICAL OR MISMATCHED breasts are far more common than most women realize. No woman has perfectly matched breasts. One is always larger than the other; one is higher than the other; one is shaped differently than the other. But while in most women this is a barely noticeable imperfection, in others it can be quite extreme.

If you are like most women reading this book, you have looked at yourself in the mirror to assess the good and bad aspects of your breasts. You may have asymmetrical breasts but not even know it. The components that contribute to asymmetrical breasts include the nipple-areola position, breast volume and shape, and skin shape and tightness. In order to evaluate whether or not your nipple-areola is in a symmetrical position, measure the distance from your sternal notch (the hollow point just below the Adam's apple) to your nipples. This measurement should be equal on both sides. You can also measure the distance from your nipple to a point on the midline of the sternum. Any difference in this measurement will result in worsening nipple asymmetry when implants are inserted.

Breast volume and shape are easier to evaluate from a purely qualitative point of view. However, to get an exact measurement of breast volume asymmetry, I suggest you use the rice test. Wearing a bra that fits your larger breast, fill the smaller breast's cup with rice in a small plastic bag until the size of both breasts looks the same. Then take the rice and pour it into a measuring cup. The milliliters on the cup is equal to the mismatch in ccs (cubic centimeters). In general, a difference between breasts of less than fifty ccs is a minimal asymmetry and in most cases does not warrant any concern. Of course, there are many women with a larger volume mismatch who are not concerned with their asymmetry and that, of course, is fine.

Skin shape and tightness will determine the overall shape and aesthetics of the breast. Asymmetry with significant skin tightness of the lower half of the breast is known as **Poland's Syndrome**, which is often the cause of the most extreme case of breast asymmetry. Medical science does not know exactly what causes Poland's Syndrome, but for some reason the embryonic blood supply is restricted on one side during an unborn infant's early development within the womb. Poland's Syndrome can have a very wide variation of results, from badly asymmetrical breasts to far more extreme problems like a deformed arm or hand on one side, or even a completely missing pectoral muscle on one side.

Even without taking Poland's Syndrome into account, there are many more women who have extremely mismatched breasts than most people realize. More importantly, most of the women who have badly mismatched breasts do not themselves realize how incredibly common it is. The reason for this is simple: The majority of women with asymmetrical breasts find the condition extremely embarrassing, so they find ways of hiding themselves from discovery. Typically, they will avoid locker rooms or any situation where they might be seen by others without a shirt on. Sometimes they go to extraordinary lengths—they might never attend physical education in school, they might never learn to swim, or they might avoid going any-place where they might be required to wear a swimsuit. In other words, they severely restrict their entire lives in order to hide their breasts. Because of this, women with mismatched breasts tend to feel very isolated and alone with their problem, not realizing that they are hiding from each other as well, and that they are in fact not alone. The feelings can be very psy-chologically damaging, and many of these women suffer from exceptionally poor self-esteem. Some never date so that they will not be "discovered." Tragically, in spite of the overwhelm-ing incidence of psychological and social distress among women with extremely mismatched breasts, insurance compa-nies very rarely cover correction of asymmetry.

Not very long ago I had a patient, an eighteen-year-old girl with asymmetrical breasts who suffered from terrible self-esteem. Painfully shy and self-conscious, she had become a virtual shut-in. Her parents were filled with worry and despair for their daughter who was preparing to go off to college without ever having kissed a boy or taken a swim with friends. A middle-class family with limited means, they petitioned their insurance company with signed letters and affidavits from psy-chologists and doctors, including myself, that this surgery was indeed a medical necessity for their daughter. In the end, they were refused and they had to borrow the money to pay for the operation. Interestingly, they came from the kind of reli-gious background where they felt that cosmetic surgery was somewhat immoral. The refusal of their insurance company to agree that the surgery was a medical necessity weighed upon them as an indictment of their motivations in helping their daughter, and they nearly decided against having the procedure done all together.

Eight weeks after the surgery, the family went on a summer vacation together. The parents were absolutely incredulous at the change that had occurred within their daughter in such a short period of time. She was a different person. She went out dancing every night, hopped into a bathing suit and went to the beach with her cousins and friends every morning, and met and dated a variety of nice young men.

When they returned to New York and their daughter came to my office for her final check up, the mother spoke to me privately and broke down in tears of gratitude for the way her daughter's life had been turned around by her surgery. There are very few moments in my career that I am more proud of, or that touched me more deeply.

The sad truth is there are many other girls out there who cannot afford this kind of surgery, and because these women with severely mismatched breasts tend to hide themselves, there will probably never be the sort of outcry necessary to create the political pressure that would force insurance companies to someday cover these procedures.

YOUR SURGICAL OPTIONS

THERE ARE SEVERAL different ways in which breasts can be mismatched, and each requires different surgical procedures for correction. A discussion of what kind of procedure you might require must begin with determining what sorts of asymmetry are present. Basically there are five factors to consider—volume, width, nipple height, height of inframammary fold, and tubular breast shape—and they may be considered alone or in conjunction with one another.

A volume asymmetry is exactly that—both breasts are

approximately the same shape and proportion, but one of them is noticeably larger in volume than the other. The simplest and most common solution to this problem is to augment the smaller breast with an implant of appropriate size. Though I very infrequently recommend the post-surgical expandable implant to my patients seeking breast augmentations, for women concerned with matching breasts that are noticeably different in volume, this can be an excellent solution. The post-surgical expandable implant has a small valve that allows the surgeon to adjust the fill level of the saline within the implant after surgery. This allows very precise control of the exact size of the implant and will allow your doctor to achieve a nearly perfect match in breast volume.

One issue that sometimes arises with volume asymmetry is when one breast, though smaller, is the same width as the larger one. If an ordinary implant is placed within the smaller breast, the width will be increased along with the size, and the patient will have exchanged a volume asymmetry for an asymmetry in shape. This can usually be solved with reasonable satisfaction by using a specially shaped implant, known as a high profile breast implant that is specifically designed to increase projection without dramatically altering the width of the breast.

There are many issues to consider when using implants for cosmetic breast surgery. For a full discussion of these issues you should read chapters four, seven, and eight.

Another frequent problem of breast asymmetry involves the height or placement of the nipple on the breast. This might or might not be accompanied by a variation in volume. The most common fix for this problem is to cut away some skin in the direction that the nipple needs to be moved (usually the lower one is raised). The nipple is then moved into position and the skin stitched in place. Though commonly used, this is not an acceptable solution. The problem is that skin is elastic by nature and merely moving the skin around without addressing the underlying structure of the breast tends to be a very short-term solution. The surgery is quick and easy, but the result is temporary because the nipple tends to slowly move back towards its original position as the skin slowly stretches. The correct way to solve this problem involves not only moving the nipple, but also performing a lift on the **parenchyma** (breast tissue) below the nipple. See Chapter Ten for more information on this surgical procedure.

Commonly, a dramatic difference in nipple height is accompanied by an asymmetry in volume. This usually requires a breast lift on one or both sides to match height and insertion of an implant on one side to match volume. Another possibility is to use two implants of different sizes to achieve the best possible result. Sometimes it may be more desirable to reduce the larger breast than to increase the size of the smaller breast, in which case there would be no need for an implant, but rather a breast lift accompanied by a reduction on one side.

Another common problem in symmetry involves the height of the inframammary fold. The inframammary fold is located at the bottom of the breast, where it attaches to the chest. It is easy to mistake an asymmetry of the inframammary fold for an asymmetry of nipple height or volume since it may appear as either of these, but the correct surgical solution may be quite different, so it is important to be able to distinguish the difference in these asymmetries.

If there is only a minor difference in the height of the inframammary fold, it may be only a minor problem in the overall asymmetry of the breast. Very satisfactory results might be obtained in this case using the techniques discussed above, such as different sized implants or breast lifts. However, if the bottoms of your breasts are attached to your chest at noticeably different heights, it will be necessary to either raise or lower one of your inframammary folds. It is generally simpler to lower the inframammary fold, but it can be tricky in some cases, especially for women with very thin or soft skin. Usually lowering the fold entails gently cutting away at the ligaments that attach the breast to the chest wall until the fold loosens a little and stretches a bit lower.

I refer to one problem that can result from this procedure as the **double bubble**. In this situation, the skin of the inframammary fold is tight enough that even though the fold is now at the correct height, the bulk of the gland tissue remains above the fold, creating a very unnatural look. This is most commonly a problem with **tubular breasts**, which I discuss in the next section.

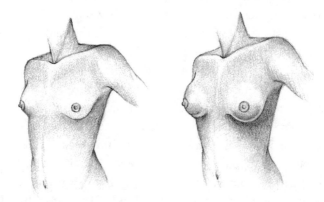

The "double bubble" phenomenon is when a tight inframammary fold is not adequately expanded during breast enlargement, thus leaving a constriction across the lower half of the breast where the old inframammary folds use to be. This is very common with tubular breast deformity.

The opposite problem sometimes occurs when lowering the inframammary fold and correcting a volume asymmetry with an implant. In patients with thin or very elastic skin, the implant, can in some cases, fall beneath the natural level of the breast, causing it to bottom out. This problem is called **implant ptosis;**

it resembles pseudoptosis in that the breast appears to sag below the nipple, causing the nipple to assume an unnaturally high position (sometimes too high to be covered by a normal bikini top). There are many ways to remedy this situation, including a procedure that I developed called an **internal physiological breast splint**. In this procedure, the natural capsule that forms around the implant is reshaped and actually used to help hold the breast and implant in position along with suturing the tissue to the chest wall. Obviously, it is best to avoid having to correct this situation, so if you have very thin and elastic skin be sure to carefully discuss the situation with your doctor.

Alternatively, in an asymmetry involving the height of the inframammary fold, it is sometimes preferable to raise one side. This slightly more complex surgery involves stitching the tissue beneath the breast higher onto the chest wall. It can be difficult to get very smooth and natural-looking results with this procedure, but sometimes the results are excellent.

TUBULAR BREASTS

THE MOST COMPLEX form of asymmetry involves tubular breasts. Tubular breasts are always a difficult situation for a plastic surgeon and they are very commonly associated with drastic mismatching of the breasts. Tubular breasts frequently involve all of the other factors mentioned in this chapter. Unfortunately, there is no way to achieve a perfect result in this situation, though a great deal of improvement may be possible.

The major challenge presented by tubular breasts is the tight and usually inflexible inframammary fold. One of the principal goals in improving the tubular deformity is to increase the width of the breast. If volume asymmetry requires an implant to correct, the tight inframammary fold will create the double bubble effect unless some additional surgical techniques are used to increase the width of the tight inframammary fold. If the tubular breast is sagging, one possible remedy is to perform a lift in addition to placing the implant. However, if there is no sagging, as in the case of some tubular breasts that project straight forward, some other technique must be used. One option is to use a tissue expander in a two-step surgery. A tissue expander is commonly used in breast reconstruction after mastectomy. This device is placed within the breast and expanded over a period of weeks in order to give the tissue a chance to stretch, expand, and actually grow. When the proper amount of tissue expansion has been achieved, a second surgery is performed to remove the expander and insert the implant. While this may seem like a great deal of effort and unpleasantness, the results are far more satisfactory than merely trying to place an implant behind a tubular breast.

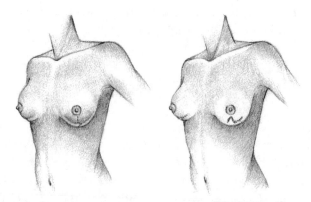

Double bubble deformity can be corrected by skin expansion or by local skin flap rotation. Here a flap of skin and soft tissue is rotated into the constricted old inframammary fold to expand it and soften the deformity.

With only a single surgery, excellent results can be achieved with this technique and it allows the patient to obtain these results. However, there may be greater scarring than with the use of the tissue expander. Both of these advanced techniques should be discussed with your doctor to ensure his or her familiarity with them. If both are equally applicable, you must weigh the benefits of a single surgery versus the additional scar of the rotation flap.

Another possibility for correcting the lack of tightness of skin in tubular breast deformity is for the surgeon to use a **rotation flap procedure**, beneath the breast where the tight fold is. In this procedure the surgeon cuts the tight fold and pulls the skin apart and outwards to either side. Then a flap of skin is lifted from below and added to the opening to allow the skin to remain apart in this more open position.

If you are a woman with mismatched breasts the main idea that I hope you take from this chapter is that you are neither alone nor unusual. As I previously stated, there are more people in your situation than you may realize. If you have the inclination, surgery can offer improvement—sometimes truly excellent improvement—for this condition.

12

Fixing Bad Surgery
For When the Unfortunate Happens

M ANY TIMES WHEN a woman comes to my office she brings a girlfriend for "moral support." On one such occasion a woman named Jeanne had come for a consultation on breast augmentation with a friend of hers who had had the procedure done herself years earlier by a different doctor. Jeanne had many excellent questions and we talked for quite a while. At some point she talked about things that might go wrong and what I could to do to prevent them. We were discussing aesthetic defects, like pectoral shelf deformity and asymmetry and the procedures that would minimize their occurrences, when suddenly, Jeanne's friend, who had been sitting quietly behind me, burst into tears and abruptly pulled her shirt off right there in my office.

Jeanne's friend, who had been happy enough with her breast augmentation to help talk Jeanne into doing it, had suddenly realized all of the things that were wrong with her own breasts. Inadvertently, I had taken a woman who was happy with her surgery and made her miserable. I felt terrible, but the truth was that she did have both pectoral shelf deformity and a high degree of asymmetry caused by a rotated anatomically shaped implant. So, I ended up with two new patients that day. Jeanne had her augmentation, and her friend decided to have revision surgery to fix the cosmetic defects from her previous surgery.

Bad surgery is most frequently not caused by bad surgeons, but by various unforeseen events and the limits of medical science to prevent every possible risk. Some bad surgery is only cosmetic, as in the case of Jeanne's friend, but sometimes it is far more serious and must be dealt with immediately.

Topping the list for fixing bad surgery are those problems that are a direct threat to the patient's health, such as infection, bleeding, or damage to the blood supply. If these types of problems are detected early, your doctor should have no problem in dealing with them. It is very important to be aware of the signs of these problems and to never be shy about discussing any fears that you might have with your doctor after (and before) your surgery. There is more information on these problems in Chapter Four, and you should be sure that you understand all of the risks and rewards. At a minimum, you should be aware of the signs of infection—fever, rash, unusual discharge—and immediately report any of these symptoms to your doctor. Being an informed patient is your best shield against risk factors.

This chapter will not deal with those types of problems because the additional surgery that they might require is not something cosmetically optional; it is, instead, something that should be taken care of immediately as a course of protecting your health. However, I would like to address some less urgent but potentially important issues that might require timely fixing. One such situation is caused by a ruptured implant. In the event that your saline implant has ruptured, the sudden deflation might be alarming, but it is not dangerous. It is, however, important to remove and replace the implant as quickly as possible—within a few days, if possible—to prevent any complications from scar tissue or closing of the pocket which contains the implant. If taken care of quickly, the replacement of an implant is simple, fast, and relatively painless.

FIXING SERIOUS CAPSULAR CONTRACTURE

ANOTHER ISSUE THAT may become necessary to deal with is advanced capsular contracture. Capsular contracture is a problem that is specifically associated with implants. So if you are considering a breast reduction or a lift that does not include an implant then this risk will not apply to you. Capsular contracture can cause a number of problems that may require revision surgery. In advanced cases the breast may take on a very round "ball" appearance. Sometimes the capsule may cause a ripple, asymmetry, or hardening that is unacceptable to you. In more serious and advanced cases of capsular contracture, you may even experience pain from the tightening of the capsule. In these cases, surgery is certainly warranted and there are several things that a surgeon can do to remedy these kinds of problems.

Usually if capsular contracture is going to be a problem, it will be obvious within the first several months of getting your implants, though sometimes it does occur much later. Depending on how advanced the capsule has become, a surgeon may opt for a **capsulotomy** or a **capsulectomy**, or even to replace the entire implant. The least invasive procedure is the capsulotomy. If you are a good candidate for this procedure, the surgeon will usually go in through the incision site to avoid further scarring and then make a few cuts in the capsule to reopen the pocket and relieve the pressure on the implant. This surgery is quick and frequently successful. Another form of capsulotomy that you may have heard of is a **closed capsulotomy**. In this procedure, the doctor does not reopen the breast at all, but rather squeezes the breast between the hands in order to "pop" the capsule open. Nobody wants additional surgery if it is not necessary, but the closed capsulotomy, in particular, has a number of serious drawbacks. Principally, the procedure may result in a ruptured implant and the manufacturers of implants not only recommend that you avoid this procedure but also consider it grounds for voiding their warrantees. Also, it is generally less effective than the open (surgical) capsulotomy, and it might be worth mentioning that many women report it to be quite painful.

A capsulectomy is a more involved surgery in which the surgeon will go in and actually remove all of the capsule tissue. Many scientists now believe that capsular contracture is caused by a micro-infection. So, after removing the capsule, the surgeon typically irrigates the entire pocket with antibiotics before reclosing the incision. As with the capsulotomy, the surgeon can generally reenter through the same incision site that was used for the initial implant procedure and thus minimize any additional scarring. Though it is a more involved and time consuming procedure with a corresponding recovery period, this is generally considered the most successful way to treat serious capsular contracture.

In most cases the surgeon will recommend that you replace the implant during a capsulectomy. This is an added level of insurance against a micro-infection sitting on the implant wall, which would cause a future problem. Since the implant hasn't ruptured and is not the direct problem, this procedure usually isn't covered by the implant warranty and, generally, the woman is required to purchase a new implant—but it is an *extremely important precaution*. One of the principal known causes of capsular contracture is micro-infection of the implant. It is extremely difficult or even impossible to remove the micro-infection from an infected implant. If the implant is not replaced during the capsulectomy, there is an increased chance that the procedure will not be successful. Therefore, it is very important that you insist on the replacement even if you must pay the additional expense for the new implant.

Another consideration when changing implants is the surface type of the implant. The implant manufacturers make both smooth and textured implants. The smooth implants are more commonly used in first-time surgeries because of the excellent aesthetic outcome. However, the smooth walled implants have a slightly higher rate of capsular contracture. In contrast, textured implants often ripple when the patient twists or turns her upper body. Therefore, after a significant capsular contracture, textured implants are the safer bet, since they add a level of security against a return of the capsular hardening.

In addition to any other treatment for capsular contracture, your doctor will probably give you a prescription for **Accolate**. This is a relatively new and not-well-understood treatment for capsular contracture, but the good news is that it does seem to work. Accolate is actually a common prescription medication for asthma. Its effect on capsular contracture was accidentally discovered when doctors noticed that some of their patients suddenly seemed to experience a dramatic reduction in previously formed capsular contracture. Why was this happening? What did these women have in common? They all had asthma, and they were all on Accolate. In subsequent studies on the effect of Accolate on capsular contracture, about 50 percent of the women involved in the study saw some improvement. In the near future we may have a better understanding of how Accolate causes this phenomenon, and be able to create better medications to prevent and relieve capsular contracture without surgery.

FIXING COSMETIC DISSATISFACTION

ASSUMING THAT YOUR cosmetic breast surgery was successful, that your recovery has gone well, and that there are no health issues relating to your surgery, the main reason that you might be considering revision surgery is that, for one reason or another, you don't like the way your new breasts look. There are many reasons why this may be so and why you might return to your doctor (or seek out a new one) to fix your previous surgery.

The first step in fixing your surgery is going to be spending some time with your doctor, determining exactly what your aesthetic deficits are and what procedures are available to remedy them. There may be only a single, simple problem or there may be many problems that you wish to address that require more elaborate surgery.

One of the most common problems that patients return for has to do with the size of their breasts. Volume issues may arise either because you want your breasts larger or smaller than they turned out or because of an asymmetry in size, and this generally will require replacing your implants with new ones or, in the case of a reduction, removing an additional volume of tissue. When it comes to volume issues, the most common request is for larger implants. Usually this procedure can be easily accomplished through the same incision site as your original surgery and the recovery is far less difficult because the pocket is already in place. The only other consideration for a woman contemplating a new implant size is that there are some studies that indicate a slightly elevated chance of capsular contracture associated with second surgery. If capsular contracture is severe, a third surgery will be required as discussed above. Given that fact, you might consider staying with the size that you have previously chosen.

There are other factors that might cause dissatisfaction, including implant movement or rotation. Rotation is a problem specific to anatomical implants since the rotation of a round implant would not be noticeable. There are two options for women who have experienced rotation of their anatomical implants. The first is to reposition them and then suture the internal tissue around them in order to better hold them in place. The other alternative is to simply replace them with round implants. This is frequently the best solution, especially for submuscular placement, where the shape of the implant is difficult to discern in any case.

If the implant has moved in some aspect other than rotation—if it has traveled higher, lower, or to either side—the problem will have to be corrected by reforming the pocket and stitching the internal tissue in place. Additionally, a self-absorbing mesh might be placed within the breast to give more support during the healing of the pocket. The most common problem with implants shifting location is when the scar tissue of the capsule has squeezed the implants higher. The best way to prevent this problem is by diligently wearing the breast band that the doctor gives you during your recovery period. Another common problem related to the trans-axillary or "armpit scar" procedure is that the implant slides down to the side, into the armpit area. All of these problems will require additional surgery to remedy and principally involve internal stitching and reforming of the pocket that holds the implants.

Where else might the implants move? **Symmastia**, also known as **bread-loafing**, is a problem where the implants have moved too far to the center. With symmastia, the implants meet in the middle, giving the appearance of a single breast in the center. The principal cause of this problem is that the surgeon cut implant pockets too close together in an attempt to create cleavage. In fact, this technique creates unnatural-looking breasts (see Chapter Two, "The Perfect Breast," for more information.). Very thin women who have very little tissue to begin with and women who have a depressed breastbone are also at additional risk. If you have a very concave chest your surgeon will likely recommend that you get a smaller implant size in order to avoid this type of complication. The surgery to fix symmastia is similar to other corrective procedures in that the pocket must be reformed and internally stitched into place. The internal scar tissue from the previous surgery might be rolled up and stitched to the chest wall to further create a barrier and a special bra will probably need to be worn during the recovery process to keep stress off the center tissue of the breast while it heals.

There are a multitude of problems associated with the transumbilical (through the belly button) insertion of implants and none of them can be corrected through the belly button—which means that all of them will require new surgery and a new scar (usually inframammary or circumareolar) to correct. One of the most pervasive problems is with the implant bottoming-out or dropping below the natural baseline of the breast. This is because the thicker skin and tissue at the base of the breast at the inframammary fold has been cut during the insertion procedure. This tissue, which normally supports the breast, is weakened and it can cause the breast to take on a dome-like and very unnatural appearance. Asymmetry is also common with this procedure. In all of these cases, correction is possible, but will require additional surgery and an additional scar. This is among the many reasons why this procedure is not recommended.

Another common aesthetic problem that is not uncommon for women who have had implant surgery is pectoral shelf deformity. This is more common with very thin women and the problem occurs when there is a lack of fullness at the top of the breast so that the implants seem to come straight out from the center of the chest like a shelf.

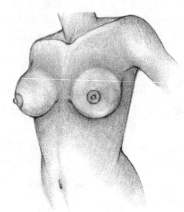

Pectoral shelf deformity occurs when the implant has an acute "take-off" from the upper chest, creating an unnatural shelf that cries, "Implants here!"

Women who have very little breast tissue to begin with and want large implants are most at risk for this kind of problem. If the implants are placed in the submuscular position this is a less common problem, though it still does occur. In this case, the remedy is to do some additional sculpting of the tissue beyond the placement of implants. The breast tissue is lifted, inside the breast and stitched to the chest wall above. If your implants were inserted from the circumareolar or inframammary position, the surgeon should be able to reenter through the same site to minimize additional scarring.

More commonly, however, pectoral shelf deformity results from a subglandular (above the muscle) placement of the implants. Less can be done in this situation because the blood supply could be compromised if the tissue is lifted after the pocket has been formed above the muscle. Aesthetic considerations are important, but safety and health always must be considered first, and it is very unlikely that a surgeon will risk compromising the blood supply in this way. The only alternative in this case is to remove the implants and reinsert them in the submuscular position. This may not completely remedy the problem, but at a minimum it will improve the situation by hiding the bulge of the implant beneath this additional amount of tissue (the muscle).

Periareolar Incision Is Your Best Option

IN VIRTUALLY every problem discussed in this chapter, the likelihood of the problem occurring would have been minimized and the repair would have been simpler if the original surgery had been performed using a periareolar incision. These are all good reasons for you to strongly consider urging your doctor to use this procedure.

FIXING SCARS

ONE OF THE MOST common secondary procedures that women return to a plastic surgeon's office for is scar revision. Plastic surgery is both an art and a science, and many techniques have been developed to minimize the appearance of scars, but it is still not possible to do surgery with no scarring at all. The incision sites are chosen to hide scars from the most casual observation and from view. Scars are made of collagen that is produced naturally by the body. The body also produces an enzyme that will slowly dissolve the excess collagen over a period of months. Usually, within six months to a year after your surgery, the scars should be faded enough to ensure very satisfactory results. But many factors affect scar formation and sometimes the scar may be darker, redder, wider, or more raised than you expected. In the worst-case scenario a keloid scar may form. Keloid scars are thick, red, and tough, and are more common on women with darker skin. There are no procedures that completely eliminate scars, but there are things that can be done to try to create thin, subtle, and barely noticeable scars.

Unacceptable scarring can be the result of many factors, including infection, smoking, excessive tension on the skin, early removal of surgical tape, improper use of ointments during the healing process, and many other unexpected events. If the cause can be isolated, it is a good signal that the revision will be more successful. Additionally, there are a number of medications, both prescription and over-the-counter, that your surgeon might recommend to prevent the excessive formation of scars or to aid your body in the reabsorption of the collagen during the healing process. More information on this topic is in Chapter Fifteen, "Taking Control of Your Recovery." It is extremely important that you don't use any medications, creams, or ointments without first checking with your surgeon. Another cause of improperly healed incision areas is the use of various products recommended by friends, herbalists, or others (even experts) without consulting your surgeon.

Finally, even in surgery where everything is as perfect as can be, there may be some kind of dissatisfaction with the appearance of your breasts. Since aesthetic satisfaction is so subjective, there is no right or wrong way for you to look. Hopefully, working with your surgeon, you can determine what course of action is best for you. As we have seen with various celebrities who have undergone countless and ever ongoing cosmetic surgical procedures, there are people who are simply never satisfied with the way they look. Perhaps this is because of an emotional dissatisfaction about themselves in general. Perhaps it is caused by something that mental health experts call **Body Dysmorphic Disorder**, the dislike of your own body regardless of how your body appears. Others suggest that for various reasons there are people who simply become addicted to plastic surgery. I am not a psychiatrist, and these issues are far beyond the scope of this book. In practice, there is almost always something that your surgeon can do to increase satisfaction with your results. If you are realistic about your goals—which is to say that what you desire is within the current abilities of the science of cosmetic surgery—there is no reason that you should not be very happy with your surgery and with your breasts.

Breast Reconstruction after Mastectomy

Repair Your Breasts and Your Self-Image!

Breast cancer is one of the most difficult experiences that a woman can endure. For some it is an attack not only on the body, but on feminine identity and self-image as well, and it can be as emotionally challenging as it is physically. Your first concern and priority in this situation must be for your health and long-term well-being. After taking all of the necessary actions to ensure your health, the consideration of whether or not to have reconstructive surgery after your mastectomy might be one of the first decisions about how you will live your life after surviving cancer.

Only you can decide if reconstruction is right for you. The arguments on each side are quite powerful, and it is particularly difficult to contemplate these issues when you are afraid for your safety and survival and your life has been turned so completely upside down. This is perhaps why, while there is very little material for women seeking *cosmetic* breast surgery in the bookstore, there are many titles available that exclusively address this issue of reconstruction. There are also many good websites that can help you through the difficult decisions in breast reconstruction. See the Internet references section at the back of this book for suggestions.

Your first consideration will be whether or not to have surgical reconstruction at all. For some women the idea of having another surgery—and the pain, recovery, and hospital time associated with it—is simply unacceptable. Breast reconstruction surgery carries all of the risks and associated problems that come with all surgeries. Beyond the risks of infection or other complications, there will certainly be swelling, additional time away from work or family responsibilities, pain, and scarring. Conversely, your oncologist will undoubtedly inform you of the many advantages of consulting with a plastic surgeon even before your mastectomy. Reconstruction allows mastectomy patients to feel more "normal" after their ordeal, more feminine, and less permanently hurt by the cancer. The missing breast for many women is a constant reminder of the fear and difficulty of dealing with cancer. Fortunately, all insurance companies are required to cover their subscribers for these procedures.

There are both emotional and physical benefits of breast reconstruction. Some women who are left with only a single breast can feel unbalanced. This applies both to the way they look and to the way they feel—the way they carry themselves in compensation for the asymmetrical weight. Long term back problems and other difficulties are associated with carrying more weight on one side of the body than the other. Many studies have been conducted that show that most women who have breast reconstruction after a mastectomy have improved mental health, a better self-image, and better sexual function than those who do not. While these studies are quite solid concerning large groups of women, it is impossible for them to predict results for any individual woman. In other words, what's right for most women might not be right for you. One thing that may help in the process of deciding is to try not to focus on what this procedure will mean to you now, but what it will mean to you for the rest of your life. How do you want to live ten or twenty years from now? After surviving your cancer you should consider that you once again have your entire life before you. You must consider your future beyond this ordeal.

RECOVERING WITHOUT RECONSTRUCTIVE SURGERY

IF YOU CHOOSE not to have any reconstructive surgery you will then decide whether to do nothing or to wear some sort of prosthesis in the place of your breast. Obviously neither of these decisions is irreversible. You may decide to go back and have reconstructive surgery at any time, even years after your mastectomy. And as to whether or not to wear a prosthesis, you may change your mind frequently and either wear or not wear one at different stages of your life.

The obvious advantages of wearing a prosthesis are that, socially, you will appear "normal" to anybody who does not know that you once had cancer, and, physically, you will not have the difficulties associated with compensating for the imbalance in weight and form of your body. Especially for women with large breasts, this can potentially save you from some serious problems with your back and neck muscles. Still, other women may be comfortable, both socially and physically, living with only one breast.

For those women who are considering a prosthesis, either permanently or until they have reconstructive surgery, Reach to Recovery, a program of the American Cancer Society, has information regarding the types of prosthetics available, where to obtain them, and how to have them correctly sized. Furthermore,

Reach to Recovery provides all women undergoing a mastectomy with a free temporary prosthesis. Reach to Recovery can be contacted at 1-800-ACS-2345.

CHOOSING RECONSTRUCTION

IF YOU PLAN to have breast reconstruction, the next decision will be whether to do it at the same time that you have your mastectomy procedure or to wait until you have recovered from the one, both physically and psychologically, before going ahead with the other. Again, the major deciding factors are both physical and emotional. The physical part of the decision is one that you can and should discuss with your surgeon. Based on your health, the procedures that you are considering, and other medical factors, your oncologist and your plastic surgeon can give you a great deal of information and perhaps even recommendations. The advantage to having both procedures done simultaneously is that you will have only one recovery period to deal with. Though that period may be lengthened and more difficult than for a mastectomy alone, it will still save a great deal of time over having the surgeries done separately. And afterwards, if all goes well, you will not have to think about the need for additional surgery in the future. This can be very compelling, but the reverse argument is that the mastectomy may be all that you can cope with at one time. Physically, you may not be up to dealing with both, and it may be easier to focus on a full recovery from your mastectomy before contemplating further surgery.

The emotional issue, as always, is more complex. For some women it is a matter of allowing themselves a period of adjustment or even grieving for the loss of the old breast before welcoming the new into their lives. Others will have the opposite response and prefer to wake up from their surgery with their new breast in place because they would prefer to never deal with being a woman without a breast. For some, the issue is about dealing with two different emotional issues at once—the emotional impact of having cancer and the emotional impact of having cosmetic breast surgery. For some women it is better to deal with both at once, while other women prefer to give each its own time. There is no "right" answer.

There are essentially two surgical options for your breast reconstruction. The first is to use implants, similar to normal breast augmentation, and the second is to reconstruct the breast using natural tissue transplanted from another part of your body. A combination of both is also not uncommon.

THE IMPLANT OPTION

FOR MOST WOMEN, the implant option will require a two-step procedure. In some cases, women with small breasts may be able to go directly to the implant in a single procedure, but after a mastectomy, most women will not have enough tissue remaining to accommodate the implant immediately. In the first procedure, the plastic surgeon will create the pocket in the submuscular position (see Chapter Seven, "Breast Enlargement.") and insert a tissue expander. The expander is like a deflated balloon with a fill valve on the front that allows the surgeon to slowly inflate it over the weeks following the initial surgery. Every one to two weeks the surgeon will add a small amount of saline with a syringe through the fill valve. This will gently cause the skin and tissue to expand until the pocket is large enough to accommodate the final implant. During this period most women report a bit of tightness or sometimes soreness immediately following each fill session. A few months after the final filling of the implant, a second surgery is scheduled and the expander is removed and the implant is placed inside the pocket.

A newer technique uses a specially made implant that also works as a tissue expander, thereby eliminating the need for an additional surgery. It works in a similar manner to the adjustable implants discussed in Chapter Seven. With the tissue expander or the single-step technique, the recovery period is ongoing during the time that the breast tissue is expanded, which may be six months or longer.

The option of using natural tissue to form the new breast is done in a single surgery but the surgery itself is much more complex and lengthy and may require a more difficult initial recovery period. The surgery may take anywhere from three to fourteen hours and usually requires a two- to four-day stay in the hospital. It may be a month or more until you can resume normal activities, such as driving, and some women report that a full return to normal activities can take six months to a year, though others report a faster recovery.

TRAM FLAP RECONSTRUCTION

THE MOST COMMON method of natural tissue reconstruction is to use tissue from the lower abdomen. This tissue, which is similar to the tissue removed in a "tummy tuck" procedure is called a **TRAM** (Transverse Rectus Abdominus Myocutaneous) **flap**, and this is the area of muscle that is taken, along with the fatty tissue above it, to form the new breast.

For some women this procedure has the added benefit of giving them a simultaneous tummy tuck. Because the tissue is taken from the lower area of the abdomen, the scar, which runs across the belly from hip to hip, will usually not be visible in normal clothing or even in a bikini, provided it doesn't have a very low-rise bottom. Once the tissue is in place, the surgeon will use the remaining natural breast as a model to sculpt the new breast as symmetrically as possible to match the original.

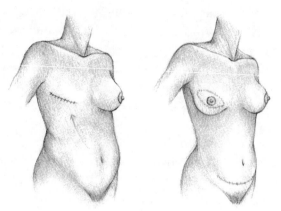

A Transverse Rectus Abdominus Myocutaneous (TRAM) flap is taken from the abdomen in order to provide additional skin and fat to the reconstructed breast. The new nipple-areolar complex is added later by tattoo or skin graft.

Aside from the mastectomy scar, which is unavoidable, the results achieved with the new breast can be very good.

There are two ways that a surgeon can move the TRAM flap from the abdomen to the mastectomy site. The more common method is to leave the tissue attached to its original arteries and veins and tunnel the whole piece through the body to the chest area. Once in place, the surgeon sculpts the tissue into a breast form and sutures the skin in place. The other method is called a "free" TRAM technique. It is called "free" because the surgeon will actually remove the piece entirely and then, using advanced microsurgery techniques, attach the flap to a new blood supply using blood vessels from beneath the arm or in the chest wall. Then the flap is attached and sculpted to the chest wall to form the breast. Some doctors prefer the free TRAM procedure because it gives them more flexibility to sculpt the breast, and they may be able to achieve a more natural-looking result. Additionally, they may want to avoid the appearance of a bulge in the abdomen that some women get from the tunneling procedure when their abdominal muscles turn upward slightly. However, there is a great deal of additional risk associated with the free TRAM technique in that if the new blood supply does not take properly, the tissue will starve and the new breast will be lost. Around 6 percent of all women will lose some small part of the new tissue, but less than 1 percent experiences a total loss of the new breast. These numbers reflect both the free, and the tunneled procedures, but overall the numbers would be slightly higher for the free. Furthermore, the tunneled or pedicle TRAM procedure is a much shorter surgery, requiring about three hours in the operating room, whereas the free TRAM procedure will require about eight to fourteen hours to complete. There are certain indications that necessitate the use of the free TRAM, including patients who are smokers, obese, diabetic, or who have scarring on their upper abdomen from previous surgeries.

There are alternative areas of the body from which your surgeon may take tissue to form the breast. The buttocks are possibilities for free flap surgery. The most common alternative site, however, is the *latissimus dorsi* muscle which runs down from the shoulder blade area of the back. This site is a very safe alternative for a tunnel procedure with very low risk to the blood supply. However, for women with large breasts it is unlikely that enough tissue can be taken from this site to match the surviving breast. In most cases, your surgeon may suggest combining a latissimus dorsi flap surgery with an implant to achieve the most natural-looking results.

The TRAM flap and other natural tissue surgeries are more serious operations with more difficult initial recovery times. They require additional and sometimes large scars. They may permanently affect your ability to perform some physical tasks (women who have had TRAM flap surgery, whether tunneled or free, report less power in the "sit-up" motion than women who have had implant reconstruction). With all of the problems associated with natural tissue reconstruction, why would you choose these techniques over the implant procedure?

The most obvious and powerful reason is that your newly reconstructed breast will be made of natural tissue. For many women the idea of having a foreign object inside their body is disturbing. Beyond the possible long-term complications relating to implants (see Chapter Four), some women simply don't like the idea that their breast is "fake." Furthermore, the overall risks associated with implants, such as the risk of severe capsular contracture, are significantly higher for breast reconstruction than for simple breast augmentation. And, of course, natural tissue looks and feels more natural. Another reason is that although the procedure is difficult and lengthy, it is a one-step process rather than the two-step process necessary for the expander and the implant. It allows the patient to wake from her mastectomy with her new breast completely in place. Another very important consideration is that, generally speaking, the TRAM flap procedure simply has better long-term results than the implant.

According to major studies, including an enormous study undertaken by the University of Michigan of women who have undergone breast reconstruction, women who have had TRAM flap procedures are more satisfied overall with their results and with the appearance of their reconstructed breasts than women who used another procedure. It turns out to be more than a matter of opinion. According to objective measurements in size, symmetry, and shape that were made during the study by the University of Michigan, breasts that have been reconstructed using natural tissue more closely match the surviving breast in every dimension studied. Because of all of these very compelling reasons, I recommend the TRAM flap surgery over implants to all of my patients for whom there is no strong medical reason against it.

FURTHER RECONSTRUCTIVE OPTIONS

THERE ARE TWO relatively new techniques in natural tissue reconstruction that are worth discussing. The first is called the **DIEP
flap procedure**. In this procedure, the plastic surgeon takes tissue from the same area of the abdomen as in the TRAM flap
procedure, except that the surgeon takes only the skin and fat,
leaving the muscle intact. The idea behind this procedure is that
by sparing the muscle, the increased risk of abdominal hernia
and abdominal weakness sometimes associated with the TRAM
surgery can be eliminated. Unfortunately, in practice, because
the procedure typically leaves some scarring on the muscle, the
abdominal wall may be left weakened very similarly to the traditional TRAM flap technique. Furthermore, this is a much more
complicated surgical technique, requiring as much as sixteen
hours in the operating room (compared with about three hours
for the TRAM procedure). And worse, this technique has a significantly higher risk of failure (flap loss). At this time, I strongly
advise my patients against this procedure.

The second new procedure is much more hopeful. It involves
a normal breast reconstruction but is done in conjunction with
something called a skin-sparing mastectomy. In the skin-sparing
mastectomy, the initial part of the surgery to remove the cancer
is done by removing the nipple, and then cutting away all of the
breast tissue inside the breast, leaving the skin intact. The TRAM
flap is then placed within the empty pocket of the breast and
fills the circle of skin left by the removal of the nipple. After nipple reconstruction this leaves virtually no serious scar, since the
border of the new nipple hides the scar. This is a simply amazing procedure. The danger associated with the procedure
involves the skin that has been spared. There is a small chance
during the mastectomy portion of the operation that some small

amount of cancerous cells will be left behind with the skin that has not been removed. This is obviously an enormous downside, but the risk for most patients is extremely low. Every case is different and the skin-sparing technique can be more or less dangerous depending upon how advanced the cancer is within the breast. Because primary concern is always for the health of the patient, this is an option that must be discussed first with your oncologist and afterwards with your plastic surgeon.

NIPPLE RECONSTRUCTION

WHICHEVER OF THESE surgeries you ultimately choose, there is one other procedure that you will probably want to consider and that is nipple reconstruction. Regardless of which procedure you use to reconstruct the breast, the reconstruction of the nipple must be done at a later date after the healing is complete. Some women do not mind the absence of the nipple, but most elect to go on and finish the job with the creation of a new nipple. Your surgeon will take some skin, usually from the reconstructed breast itself and shape it into a cone to form the new nipple. Additional tissue may be taken, usually from the site of the mastectomy scar or the edge of the scar from the TRAM flap procedure (if there is one), to form the areola. The reconstructed nipple will be the same color as the surrounding skin and many women will eventually have a tattooing procedure to match the color of their other nipple. Both the reconstruction and the tattooing involve very little if any discomfort since the nerves of the reconstructed breast may be numb.

Another good technique which may be available to you for nipple reconstruction uses the opposite areola (of the surviving breast) to make a perfect match. This may be done in cases where the patient has a lift or reduction of the surviving breast in order to match the new breast.

INSURANCE

THE WOMEN'S HEALTH and Cancer Rights Act of 1997 made it possible for any woman with health insurance, even managed care programs, to have breast reconstruction following a mastectomy. This is a very positive and compassionate piece of government legislation that guarantees that your health care provider will pay for your reconstruction in any way that you and your doctors decide is best for you. In other words, no insurance plan may limit your choice of procedures. Furthermore, they are also required to pay for any cosmetic surgery on the surviving breast, if you and your doctor deem it necessary to achieve symmetry and aesthetic matching with your reconstructed breast. For example, if a woman wishes to have a natural tissue reconstruction but does not have enough tissue in her TRAM flap area to create a large enough breast to match her surviving breast, she may opt to have the surviving breast reduced or lifted to create matching, natural-looking breasts.

Breast cancer is a terrible disease that still kills many women every year. But if detected early, there is no reason that you cannot survive this disease, and with plastic surgery, there is no reason that this disease should prevent you from having the most normal and happy life possible afterwards. As a plastic surgeon, my most fervent hope for my reconstruction patients is that ten years from their surgery, deeply involved in their normal lives, they never have occasion to even think about me or that small, scary time in their past that brought them to my office.

The Psychology of the Breast

A Look at the Psyche of a Society Fixated on Breasts

By Jennifer N. Duffy, PhD, Clinical Psychologist

A S A PRACTICING clinical psychologist for the past twelve years, I have had many patients come to my office with complaints and concerns that revolved around self-image and their bodies. I have also had the pleasure of appearing on many talk shows (Geraldo, Ricki Lake, Sally Jesse Raphael, and others) to discuss this same problem. I was originally consulted on this book to help Dr. Freund explain the complex psycho-social considerations of the breast, and why they are so important in our society. During our discussions, Dr. Freund decided that it would be best for me to write this chapter to help you unravel the complex tangle of emotions that surround the psychology of the breast.

When we hear the term "plastic surgery" what comes to mind is the physical material that we might imagine is used in producing plastic or silicone. In reality we get the term "plastic" from the Greek word *plastikos* which means "to mold or give form to." Plastic surgery gives new form to the body and with that new form comes a new mental body image. Hopefully, this new body image is the image that surgery was chosen to create.

There are always mental and emotional consequences to any surgery. Those associated with cosmetic alterations can be profound, as the sole reason most people choose to undergo the procedure is to augment both their breasts and their self-esteem. If a desired surgical change in appearance does not come about just as you had envisioned in your mind's eye, emotionally devastating results can occur. Although it is human nature to seek perfection in an imperfect world, many times disappointment can be the result of attempting to "improve" the physical attributes that God and D.N.A. have bestowed upon us. More important, however, is the very real fact that there is no "magic bullet" to improve interpersonal relationships or solve all of our problems. If a patient is genuinely unhappy with herself and her life, undergoing breast augmentation or reduction is not going to change these unfortunate facts. We live in a push-button society of instant gratification where we wait for nothing. Fast food, microwaves, fax machines, credit cards, email, cell phones, and even psychotropic medication all give us what we want very quickly and with very little effort. Therefore, we as a society have become accustomed to seeking these types of solutions to our problems. The important thing to remember is that plastic surgery is not a quick fix for a poor self-image or lack of self-esteem. It is really only effective in *enhancing*, not creating those essential aspects of a well-adjusted personality.

The purpose of this chapter is to assist you in engaging in a process to help you make the very profound decision as to whether or not to attempt a cosmetic surgical breast augmentation or reduction. Our society's fascination with large breasts and how they impact self-esteem, mental body image, femininity, and even self-worth will be addressed. There is the expression that, "It is a man's world." This implies that men hold all the power in our society. However, we might have to recognize that in many instances, "It is a young, beautiful, well-endowed woman's world." Big tits are powerful. They attract and often get the attention of males who just might give up a lot in order to get ahold of them.

FROM NURTURE TO SEX OBJECT

PRIMARILY, THE GREATEST function of the breasts is to feed a child. This has evolutionary significance in that, long before Enfamil and Similac, mother's milk was the only means of sustaining an infant's life. Breasts have always had a prominent role in human existence and are valued for that reason. Colostrum—the mother's antibodies that are transferred to the newborn through suckling—take on essential significance in immunizing the child against disease during the first two days of life prior to the production of milk. An infant makes certain antibodies but can get others only from its mother during this critical period of life. Even the term "nurturing," which today connotes all things important in rearing a child, is derived from the Latin root *nutrire* which means "to provide with substances necessary to life and growth." Two instincts that an infant is born with are rooting and suckling. Therefore, a baby is preprogrammed to know that it has to draw on his or her mother's breast for survival. That is a powerful innate force. While the baby suckles, it is fed, but also engendered with a sense of comfort, tranquility, and security that is pure. Forever after in life a human will try to recapture that profoundly content state of being. These are some of the reasons we as a society are preoccupied with the breasts whether we were breast-fed or not.

Although the breasts have a nuts and bolts physical function, over time they have become sex objects. The breasts, and more specifically the nipples, are known as one of the erogenous zones of the body. Fondling them and caressing them stimulates the sexual response. For many women they are a significant source of both sexual pleasure and elicit other bodily processes which ready the woman for intercourse. This leads to gratification on an individual level yet also provides for propagation of the species. Sex, aside from reproduction, facilitates bonding within a relationship, creates intimacy, and is a tremendous outlet for stress. The sex drive is an innate human instinct that motivates behavior and must have an outlet. Not having intercourse on a regular basis can lead to pent up feelings that manifest themselves as frustration, irritability, anger, depression, agitation, or anxiety. These emotions make people sad and put them in psychic pain. That is why the breasts are vital to a woman's psychological health.

NATURE VERSUS NURTURE

BODY IMAGE AND self-esteem begin to develop almost from birth, long before we are aware of the influences of the media and society at large. Research studies have clearly shown that parents treat boy babies differently than girl babies. Specifically, little boys are perceived as tougher and are traditionally interacted with in a rougher, more playful fashion. Little girls are traditionally considered more delicate and treated much more gently. Additionally, little girls are often dressed in gender specific clothing, such as pink dresses, bows, and hats. This socialization process also extends to the toys that are presented to very young children. Whereas little boys are typically given trucks and GI

Joes, little girls are typically showered with baby dolls and Barbies. Interestingly, studies have shown a gender specific preference for very young children to gravitate towards traditionally "same sex" toys. There is an age-old psychological debate of "nature versus nurture." Are we who we are because of the influence of genetics or is it environment? In answering this question of what dictates stereotypical behavior, as usual, the answer is that it is a combination of both.

When it comes to the influence of nurture or environment on the development of a little girl's perception of the "typical" female form, we need to look no further than the toys that they are given as young as the age of two or three. Aside from their mothers or other significant female caregivers they may be exposed to, little girls are often presented with a Barbie or similar doll that is "anatomically correct" right down to her full bosom, small waist, and full hips. During this stage of imaginary play, this is the image that little girls not only identify with, but also aspire to be like when they grow up. In addition to toys, one needs only to think of the influence of pictorial representations of iconic fairy-tale heroines such as Cinderella, Snow White, and Sleeping Beauty. Even Mr. Purity, Walt Disney, gave these characters big breasts. These classic stories all depict the young women as beautiful, sweet, and ultimately getting the men of their dreams and living happily ever after. This is a powerful message to send to a child and over time becomes internalized in that these characteristics become associated with the attainment of these fantasies. Many women aspire to this "idyllic fairy-tale existence" into adulthood, where they strive to find their Prince Charming, live in a castle, have beautiful little children, and possess a perfect body.

After the influence of young childhood comes the effects of puberty that is signaled by the development of secondary sex characteristics, the most objectively noticeable of which is the emergence of a girl's breasts. At a glance, breasts are what distinguish a woman from a man. It is the most superficial way a woman can identify with her femininity. This occurs at different ages depending on genetics and diet. Yet it is also occurring at a very critical and fragile time emotionally, a time when fitting in and looking like your friends is of the utmost importance. A pecking order is established—who's ahead, who's behind, who's big, and who's small. These differences begin to take on importance just when the dynamics of social interaction are changing. Specifically, girls ages five to eleven leave the latency stage that, according to Sigmund Freud, is an asexual period that involves predominantly same sex interactions of a nonsexual nature. Involvement with the opposite sex is limited and often avoided. However, once a girl enters the genital stage (age eleven to adulthood), interest in the opposite sex is awakened. It is at this point that a young girl begins to become aware of her sexuality and seek out interactions with the opposite gender that are of a sexual nature. It is here that young women begin to experience firsthand the value and importance of breast size.

Those girls who develop early and abundantly become the most sought after and popular in terms of the amount of attention they receive from many males. A normal, emotionally well-adjusted adolescent male is likely to get his first impression of the All-American Girl's physical form by examining *Playboy* magazine or some similar source. Let's be honest: Pick up any issue of *Playboy* and you won't find one A-cup. Such images burn deeply into the consciousnesses of horny young men who no doubt have their first powerful masturbatory experiences while gazing at them. These first ejaculations cause nervous impulses to register vivid "memories" in the limbic system, or pleasure center of the brain. To recreate a sexual high of the same intensity, similar or more archetypical images must often be used. When a real woman's form usually does not measure up to what has been associated with such profound feelings of joy, disappointment and unattainable expectations can ruin what should be normal sexual interactions for a lifetime.

From a behavioral standpoint, any cues that are present in these first male sexual experiences become conditioned stimuli, meaning they are associated with arousal and over time the presentation of them alone can elicit the sexual response. Lingerie, high-heeled shoes, female body parts like the breasts, legs, or buttocks, all become sexualized objects due to their frequent pairing with sexual stimulation. Depending upon what a man typically focuses on, this sexualized object becomes his primary source of arousal. This explains why some men define themselves as "breast men."

It seems guys have segregated themselves into one of four categories: breast men, butt men, leg men, and face men. These categories denote the singular aspect of a woman that they value most and seek out in a mate. Some men relate a common modus operandi of focusing on a woman in large gathering places like a party, club, or bar. The crowd is scanned to pick out female candidates with one of these four singular superficial qualities that the individual guy feels he needs most. When he zeros in on a girl with those goods, he goes over to initiate conversation and discover if she has the other deeper attributes he also desires, like intelligence, being a good conversationalist, or having a good sense of humor. Pirandello in his play *The Naked* said, "The bait of appearance masks the hook of reality." The bottom line is that some men won't even look at you unless you have big tits. Now, if you want to play that game, so be it. Just understand what you are doing and why you are doing it. If you want to be a target for a breast man in a bar you will get them all: the good, the bad, and the ugly. So be prepared with a few verbal zingers with which to defend yourself.

Breasts in Art History

SO WHAT are the roots of modern culture's obsession with big breasts? If we examine classic Renaissance artwork, such as Botticelli's "The Birth of Venus," in the context of the accepted modern aesthetic, these are paintings of "fat" women. Yet, in the age when these works were created, being "overweight or voluptuous" was an outward sign to the world that you were well fed and opulent, even powerful. Botticelli's goal was to depict a living "goddess of love," not some scrawny undernourished common woman. It could be here that the notion of "big is better" was first disseminated by the mass media of the times: oil painting. Wealthy patrons paid great artists to capture, on canvas and in stone, the likeness of their wives, concubines and courtesans. All of these ladies, through the generosity of their powerful protectors, were well cared for and had more than enough to eat, which made them appear curvaceous and develop large breasts.

THE INFLUENCE OF POPULAR CULTURE

AS TIME HAS evolved, we as a society have evolved as well in terms of what we value when it comes to the female form. Television is the main medium that children are exposed to. For many it substitutes for their baby-sitter. We grow up with this companion that becomes our primary source of information but also our main conduit of information flow and our window on the world. The average person does not question what is presented but instead accepts what he or she sees as an accurate reflection of true existence. Gone are the days of reading or listening to the radio for information and entertainment. Instead, people are tuned into attractive talking heads that read them the news. Turn on any television show and you will see that the majority of the actors are young, attractive, and in great shape.

The biggest complaint of actors is that there aren't enough roles for aging stars. This presents a slanted view of the human experience to all people, young and old. Yet it is one that we all want to emulate. A *Time* magazine article from the late 1970s stated that, "Television is the mental static that distorts our view of reality and ourselves."

We are a beauty- and youth-driven society and that has its consequences, one of them being the popularity of cosmetic surgery. Liz Taylor had a major face-lift, which was documented in the movie *Ash Wednesday* in the late 1960s. This caused a sensation at the time not only because it was such a radical and extreme notion to use a scalpel and cut your face to achieve a more youthful look, but to make public that she had it done. However, fast-forward thirty years and stars are being featured on the covers of magazines proudly discussing their latest cosmetic enhancement. Cosmetic surgery is no longer taboo, and it isn't just for the rich and famous anymore. People in their thirties, as opposed to their sixties, are now beginning to obsess about the aging process and slowing it down. This is indicative of how we've been indoctrinated by what television shows us to the point where it affects what we value and ultimately alters our behavior.

Fashion and cosmetics are multibillion dollar industries. They've paid advertising gurus fortunes to influence our buying practices. The designers and fashion magazine editors dictate what we wear and how our clothes should fit. Every magazine cover or advertisement features a young, beautiful, well-endowed model. We are so obsessed with selling and achieving perfection that the pictures of all of these gorgeous creatures, these supermodels, are airbrushed. Yet to the public, this is not obvious. It only reinforces the belief that it is possible to look this way. Yet because no one really does, we have to seek unnatural solutions to try to achieve this ideal. We as a society like pretty things. We all want to look in the mirror and see an attractive image staring back so we can feel pretty. If we didn't value appearances, people wouldn't put themselves through the physical torture of exercise and the deprivation of dieting.

Music is another medium that influences people, both young and old. Gone are the days when a singer only had to have a good voice to be a star. Tune into MTV and you will see that this is true. We are bombarded with images of Britney Spears and Beyoncé, both of whom can not only carry a tune but are beautiful, scantily clad, and very sexy. This too has a profound impact on girls, who want to be like them in every way.

Due to this dynamic of human experience involving the breasts, a inadequacy can develop. Such manifest feelings of insecurity and poor self-image can affect a woman for the rest of her life. A good friend of mine was tall, thin, and flat-chested as a girl. I had only come to know her when she was in her late twenties and was a stunningly beautiful, vivacious woman. She had a great body that could stop traffic yet inside, just below the surface, she saw herself as Olive Oil. That stinging moniker, given to her by a cruel female classmate, had been so emotionally devastating that, despite the fact she was a late bloomer who ultimately blossomed incredibly well, it had skewed her self-image.

NEEDS, BEHAVIOR, AND BREASTS

WHEN YOU ARE an adolescent and find your friends' breasts develop more rapidly than yours, all kinds of societal pressures can cause you to take matters into your own hands. "Stuffing," the "Wonder Bra," even gel inserts are all well and good, but what do you do when the clothes come off? This type of behavior only lends itself to further potential social humiliation and self-image issues, yet lays the groundwork for the desire to seek a more permanent and natural solution.

Breast augmentation and reduction can be considered a form of "self-mutilation" in that the skin is cut, the body reshaped, and residual scarring is left, whether large or small. This, in conjunction with all the potential risks discussed in this book, may leave many people wondering why a woman would ever consider going under the knife to begin with. It is really quite simple when you look at it from a behavioral perspective. Specifically, needs are what drive an individual's behavior. We all can have multiple needs at the same time, but it depends upon which need takes number one importance that ultimately determines the behavior an individual exhibits. For example, in my daily private practice I have many patients that come in expressing a desire to be happy. Yet we know from research studies that most people don't change. Your own interpersonal experience may have shown you this. That is because although many people have a need to be happy, they also have a need to be comfortable. Change creates anxiety, which is unpleasant. Most people are unwilling to tolerate the anxiety of change, even if temporary, due to their primary need to be comfortable. So although an individual may be unhappy, there is a certain predictability and safety in knowing that tomorrow you will be just as unhappy as you are today. To try and achieve happiness, one must take a chance and enter a world of unknowns that disrupts this feeling of comfort, which for many people is their number-one priority. As long as this order remains, a person will never achieve happiness because he or she will be unable to take the necessary steps to accomplish it. This is a sad but true commentary of human nature.

Women who ultimately seek out plastic surgery have reached a point in their lives where they have become most uncomfortable with their appearance and the way it makes them feel about themselves. Although they may be fearful of the potential side effects, like loss of breast sensitivity or complications of surgery, in their hierarchy of needs, a desire to be happy with the way they look and feel and reap all the anticipated rewards associated with the desired results has taken priority. This need to change their breasts is what will ultimately drive and determine their behavior.

In addition to being reminded of the possible negatives, patients are also informed of the thousands of women who have this procedure done every year with relatively few problems. Therefore, if what is most important is to achieve an ideal body image and rid oneself of this discomfort, a woman will mentally downplay her fears regarding the risks and instead focus on the positives to ultimately achieve her goal.

WEIGHING RISKS AND REWARDS

SURGERY IS SURGERY. Surgery is no joke. There is no such thing as "simple" or "routine" surgery. Making an informed decision before undergoing any procedure involves understanding all of the possible things that could go wrong and an ultimate acceptance of those risks. The lengthy disclaimer that each patient must sign presupposes that she has duly researched and understood the specialized knowledge involved. Aiding that process is the purpose of this book and specifically this chapter. It is important to remember that the process of weighing risks and rewards is a personal and relative one, and should result in a decision that you make on your own, for yourself.

Any normal, emotionally well-adjusted patient should have a palpable fear of a scalpel cutting through her flesh. Scarring of the breast tissue is an inexorable consequence of that incision. This may alter a woman's self-image and ultimate satisfaction with the procedure. Push-up bras and gel inserts can achieve the same look in clothing that a more radical surgery would without the same risks. So the general public doesn't have to know how you achieved that perfectly proportioned body, especially if it is only temporary. Ironically, the only person who would perceive you differently and ever view the inevitable scarring, whether major or minor, is the person you are most intimate with. Theoretically, that is the person you care most about in life and whose opinion on your appearance is most valued. In addition, this is the individual you want to ultimately sexually excite but who may be turned off by the scarring or even the notion your breasts are "fake."

The cutting edge of a scalpel blade could also interfere with the nervous impulses that generate feelings of sexual excitation from the erogenous zone of the nipple. If you are considering this procedure, you should think long and hard about how you would cope with the loss of this mechanism were it to be permanent. This is a true potential side effect of any augmentation or reduction surgery, though in many instances this loss of feeling is only temporary. You need to weigh the importance of this major source of sexual gratification with your desire to have nicer looking breasts that are potentially numb.

Due to the potential loss of nipple sensation that may or may not ever return, many people might question why a woman would want to risk losing this significant source of erotic stimulation and pleasure. The answer for many women who are dissatisfied with their breasts is that they never liked having them touched to begin with due to overwhelming feelings of self-consciousness. So, yes, their breasts are an erogenous zone, but the psychological shame, embarrassment, and feelings of inadequacy may have kept the nervous system connections from functioning properly anyway. The trade-off of potentially losing "feeling" yet gaining the self-perception that one is and "feels" sexier is a no-brainer.

As most people learn sooner or later, sex is 80 percent mental and 20 percent physical. Even though you may be physiologically capable of arousal through stimulation, whether or not you seek it out or actually enjoy it depends highly on your mood state and psychological frame of mind. This is truer for women then it is for men. Men are very visually oriented. All it takes is a little eye candy to get them aroused, whereas with women our emotions play a big role in setting the stage for sexual interactions. Specifically, we are more sensitive to the way we feel about ourselves and our mates when it comes to wanting and pursuing sex. If we feel depressed, self-conscious, or insecure about our partners, we are less likely to get aroused. The drive for sex is thought to be a primary drive that motivates our behavior. So it is not surprising that the desire to be and feel sexy can impel a woman to take measures that would appear to the average individual to be drastic.

Another fear associated with cosmetic breast surgery is the potential interference of the implants with the ability to breast-feed a baby. As we discussed, suckling is a tremendously rewarding experience for both infant and the mother. There is no more natural and beautiful bonding experience that a woman can share with her child then to continue nourishing it from her body beyond birth. There is a certain sense of loss, as strange as this may sound, that a woman feels after giving birth. In extreme cases this can contribute to postpartum depression. Breast-feeding prolongs this psychic and physical connection and diminishes these feelings of loss. Anyone can change a diaper or give a bottle; only a mother can feed her child in this way. The fear of the potential disruption of this uniquely female experience is understandable. Therefore, it is important to discuss this issue with your surgeon.

CHANGING FROM THE INSIDE OUT

HUMAN BEINGS SEEK perfection in an imperfect world. This is a fool's game that no one ever wins. Instead of buying into the collective lie of looking a certain way in order to feel a certain way, one should work from the inside out. Specifically, it is important to learn to value yourself for other qualities besides those that are purely physical. Logically, age wins out. We all rot a little bit every day, ultimately sag, wrinkle, and become dust. Aging is an inexorable process that cannot be prevented. You should take these statements to heart because even if you elect to have cosmetic surgery, these are still facts that you ultimately have to face.

Lack of self-esteem is the primary factor that leads to dissatisfaction and psychological disorders. Because self-esteem is an internal mechanism, it can only be adjusted from the inside out. Specifically, you need to learn to like and value yourself for the things that make you unique as opposed to emphasizing the qualities you dislike in yourself. We all have strengths and weaknesses. No one is perfect. However, what you choose to focus on at any given moment will dictate how you feel. We've all had the experience of getting a new haircut. Nine people may say they like it and one person does not. Yet it is a common human failing to focus and give more importance to this one negative opinion as opposed to the nine positive reactions you received and ultimately feel bad about your new look. Thoughts are habits. It takes practice to train yourself to think differently, focus on different things, and value yourself in other ways. Often a professional, depending on the ingrained nature of this thought pattern, can facilitate this task. As the popular saying goes, "To dream of the person you'd like to be, is to waste the person you are." If you are considering breast augmentation or reduction in order to become "the person you'd like to be," don't even consider it until you have seen a therapist in order to work on "the person you are."

That's not to say that you shouldn't care about your appearance and completely let yourself go. Taking pride in the way you look is indicative of how you care about yourself. However, all behavior is neither good nor necessarily bad, but often is a matter of degree. It is extremely important to be realistic in your expectations about yourself, your appearance, and what it can do for you. If the only thing that matters to you is your exterior and most of your day is spent focused on that, then you will most certainly neglect your intellect and your personality and all that those things have to offer. These inner qualities ultimately attract people to us and are what make us valued as individuals. It is therefore important to give significant attention to developing those inner qualities we have that make us special, as they are not only enduring, but, whether we realize it or not, we also have much more control over them. Making yourself better inside will lend itself to a more real change in self-image and ultimately self-esteem.

QUESTIONS YOU SHOULD ASK YOURSELF

FOLLOWING ARE A LIST of questions you should ask yourself when making the decision as to whether or not you should seek breast reduction or augmentation. It is important to really search your soul and be honest with yourself as this is a relatively permanent solution that can have far-reaching effects on your life and your self-image.

1. Am I about to cosmetically enlarge or reduce my breasts primarily for myself and not just for someone else?
2. Do I understand that flesh is not clay and perfection does not exist in this world?
3. Do I know that all surgery has potential side effects?
4. Have I educated myself of the side effects and success rate of the surgical procedure I am considering and accepted those potential risks?
5. Are larger or smaller breasts something that I have always wanted?

6. Do I feel that altering my breasts will help me feel sexier and more confident?
7. Do I feel that altering my breasts will augment my self-esteem, but not magically create it?

If you answered yes to the above questions, then chances are you have seriously weighed the pros and cons of plastic surgery, are realistic in your expectations, and are probably doing it for the right reasons. If you are wavering on some or all of those questions, then it would be wise to wait to make this decision and discuss it further with a mental health professional.

REASONS *NOT* TO HAVE COSMETIC SURGERY

FOLLOWING IS A LIST of the wrong reasons for undergoing plastic surgery of *any* kind. If you answer yes to one or more of these questions, then it is quite likely that you have underlying issues that need to be addressed with a professional. Undergoing surgery without resolving these problems will affect your expectations going in, your perception coming out, and ultimately your satisfaction with yourself and the procedure. This is too serious an issue to take lightly. Waiting and processing your motivations and potential underlying problems in therapy can not only prevent you from making a mistake but will only improve your life and possibly achieve what you are hoping surgery will. Either way, therapy is a win-win situation with minimal consequences, unlike surgery with all of its risks.

Are you expecting that breast augmentation/reduction will . . .

1. make your spouse desire you more?
2. get you more attention from men?
3. solve marital or relationship problems?

4. create self esteem?
5. make you less depressed?
6. make you lose weight?
7. make you exercise regularly?
8. heal emotional scars?
9. exact revenge against people who teased you?
10. bring you happiness?
11. bring you love?
12. make you feel like a female idol?
13. get you Mr. Right?
14. get you laid?
15. get you a better orgasm?
16. get you a husband?
17. keep your husband?
18. make you powerful?
19. give you an opportunity for men to get to know the real you?

REAL STORIES FROM WOMEN WHO HAVE HAD COSMETIC BREAST SURGERY

FOLLOWING ARE TRUE accounts of real cosmetic surgery patients of Dr. Freund who have had either a breast augmentation or a breast reduction. These women have agreed to share their experiences, both good and bad, as a way of enlightening those who are considering a similar procedure. It is certainly one thing to read a clinical description of a surgical intervention and quite another to understand firsthand the motivations for undergoing one and the psychological results that you can expect. Unless you have a good friend who has had her breasts enhanced or reduced, it is difficult and awkward to approach a woman to find out what her real experience was both before and after. Therefore, in reading these women's accounts you may find that you identify with their feelings and it may also help you to develop more realistic expectations as you read how surgery did and did not change their lives.

In speaking with these patients, the overwhelming reason why they sought out plastic surgery was to enhance a healthy sense of self-esteem. Interestingly and significantly, they report that they *already possessed a positive self-image.* They did not undergo surgery to create self-esteem or fix the problems that they had in their lives. In addition, they all concurred that they did this for *themselves,* despite positive or negative feedback they may have received from their friends and families. Therefore, their experiences were relatively positive because they were realistic in their expectations and underwent the procedure for the right reasons. Additionally, they also chose the right surgeon, which is critical to obtaining good results. It should be noted that this is not a representative sample of women who have undergone mammoplasty, and their experiences may not be typical of all surgical patients. Rather, it is meant to give the reader some insight into what these women went through, in their own words, and how it did or did not change their lives.

Most interesting to me is these women's belief that the development of an ideal breast size is solely an internal process without the impact of any external influence. However, they all acknowledged that they never looked the way that they wanted to in clothes or lingerie. The design, manufacturing, and advertising of clothing is certainly an external factor that is influenced or created by the fashion industry which has an obvious prototype for whom it designs clothing—thin women with full breasts, small waists, and full hips. If the average female consumer wants to look the way a model appears in a print ad and fill out the clothing in the appropriate places, then she is forced to wear padded bras or seek more permanent solutions such as plastic surgery. They all said that a certain size was most in proportion to their bodies, which is why it was chosen by them and their surgeon. In addition, they all voiced great satisfaction with the clothing they could now wear and the joy in going into a store and being able to buy clothes that fit them the way they wanted them to. This indicates that we as women are driven by our own internal prototype that is shaped by external factors, whether we realize it or not. These influences could be the shape of the clothing we buy, the magazines we read, the TV shows and movies that we watch, all of which contain thousands of images of what society deems to be attractive. We are exposed to these factors from the time we are aware of our surroundings to the day we die. Of course, this is often a passive, subconscious process that we are unaware of, but it definitely affects how we see ourselves as well as how we feel about the way we look.

NAME: Ann
PROCEDURE: Breast reduction
BRA SIZE BEFORE: 40 EE
BRA SIZE AFTER: 36 C
AGE WHEN SURGERY WAS PERFORMED: 56
CURRENT AGE: 57
MARITAL STATUS: Widowed 4 years
OCCUPATION: Marketing
HIGHEST LEVEL OF EDUCATION: Master's degree
NUMBER OF CHILDREN: 0

Ann's primary motivation for having breast reduction surgery was borne of the belief that her chronic back pain and osteoarthritic knees were a result of postural imbalances caused by her overly large and weighty breasts. This was compounded by her inability to exercise consistently or get into shape, as doing so would aggravate her back pain. The only exercise that she could tolerate was swimming, but she felt too self-conscious in a swimming suit to do it often. Even more frustrating was the fact that no matter how much she dieted and exercised, she was unable to lose weight in her chest. Ann's orthopedic surgeon concurred that surgery would help to alleviate her pain.

Though she described herself as a confident, successful woman, Ann's self-consciousness manifested itself in the fact that she never wanted her picture taken, or if she did she made sure to stand behind someone to hide the size of her breasts. She would wear baggy clothing to camouflage herself and avoided looking in a mirror because it made her feel sad. Ann was adamant that she had surgery only for herself and did not even tell her boyfriend until the surgery was scheduled.

Following her reduction procedure, Ann began to exercise three to four times per week with no pain whatsoever. She has continued this lifestyle change to this day and has lost a total of forty-five pounds since her surgery. She most enjoys the ability to go clothes shopping, as she will now actually look in the mirror when she tries something on. Ann is now wearing clothes that are sexier, with plunging necklines that she never would have worn before. This has had a positive effect on her self-image in that she feels great about herself and has more confidence in her appearance. It is important to reiterate, however, that before her surgery Ann described herself as a confident person.

The surgery had no impact on Ann's sex drive, but she now feels less self-conscious about her breasts. Her boyfriend did admit that he was initially attracted to her because of her large breasts, but he is happy with the results because of how happy and satisfied Ann is, not to mention that he thinks she looks great.

Ann also noted that most people don't realize she had the procedure done. They just notice that she looks great—younger, thinner, and much happier—which she would certainly agree with. She never had difficulty attracting men, who continually tell her how good she looks instead of ogling her breasts. Women are more curious about the surgery itself. Her biggest complaint was that she let someone talk her out of having her breasts reduced ten years ago. In addition, many people will ask her if she plans to undergo additional cosmetic procedures, to which she responds by using sarcasm, as she has no intentions of doing anything else.

Most important was Ann's intention of following through with the procedure despite the potential negative reactions of others. She did this strictly for *herself*. Ann would not only go through this procedure again, but would also recommend it to others. Ann reported that her doctor, Dr. Freund, was very thorough in preparing her, so she did not have any preconceived ideas about the outcome. The confidence he instilled in her before and after helped her to overcome her primary fear of general anesthesia.

NAME: Gay
PROCEDURE: Breast augmentation with a lift
BRA SIZE BEFORE: 34 B
BRA SIZE AFTER: 34 D
AGE WHEN SURGERY PERFORMED: 44
CURRENT AGE: 45
MARITAL STATUS: Married 8 years to second husband
OCCUPATION: Homemaker
HIGHEST LEVEL OF EDUCATION: High school, 2 associates' degrees
NUMBER OF CHILDREN: 4

Gay stated that her main reason for having breast augmentation stemmed from always having been self-conscious about her body. She has always exercised and taken care of herself; however, the stigma of being a chubby child has stayed with her throughout adulthood. At the age of thirty, following the birth of her first child, Gay began to feel uncomfortable with her breasts. She attributed this to having a larger bustline during her pregnancy, which had made her more comfortable with her appearance. This, coupled with the effects of gravity, made her seriously consider surgery after the birth of her third child four years ago. In addition, Gay reported that as a dedicated mother who raised her children alone until she remarried, she felt that she had never done anything for herself and felt it was finally time to do so. Although she did this for herself, her husband was very supportive, and in some ways she did it for him as well. After a few months of contemplating her options, Gay made the decision to have the procedure.

Following her surgery, Gay was very swollen and had to wear large bras that prevented her from wearing normal clothes. Although this made her feel somewhat fat, it was only temporary. Otherwise it was not obvious that she had had anything done, so she did not feel too uncomfortable around others. Once the healing was over she was satisfied with the natural look and feel of her breasts, which are now proportioned exactly as she wanted them to be. Regarding feelings of dissatisfaction, she reported none and says that she did not experience any loss of nipple sensation, which had been a concern for her.

Gay has always gotten attention from both sexes, the only difference being that now she gets more. She stated that at her age the only things her breasts are good for is making her feel attractive to others and feel good about her self. Although she is happily married and not looking to attract another mate, she enjoys the way positive male attention enhances her self-esteem. She mentioned that it also makes her husband feel proud, which she attributes to her belief that all men are teenagers at heart.

Gay's friends were also very supportive of her decision. She decided not to tell her parents until after the fact as she knew they wouldn't have approved of elective surgery and did not want to deal with the potentially negative feedback. Afterwards, it was never really discussed, but she believes that they are happy as long as she is happy.

Conversely, Gay's teenage children initially had a primarily negative reaction. At the time of her surgery her son was almost fifteen, and her daughter was twelve, both difficult ages in terms of emotions and self-esteem. Gay's decision to undergo breast augmentation became a huge source of embarrassment for them after their friends and other parents started gossiping. Furthermore, her daughter had a lot of difficulty coping because she was a female just entering adolescence and beginning to experience self-image issues of her own. Gay dealt with these adverse reactions by recognizing that teenage children often feel embarrassed by their parents as a part of their normal development, so some of the negative feelings would have likely occurred anyway. A year since the surgery, her kids now feel more comfortable with her and her decision.

Overall, Gay is proud of herself for enjoying her results and not allowing herself to experience any regrets. Due to the very positive experience of her first cosmetic surgery and the way it impacted on her self-esteem, Gay later elected to undergo abdomenoplasty (a tummy tuck) to correct the scarring and distortion to her body from three pregnancies and caesarean births.

Due to her positive experience, Gay reported that she would absolutely go through her breast augmentation procedure again and would definitely recommend it to others. This experience has only enhanced the way she feels about herself. She feels as if she is twenty again, only better. Because she had lost thirty pounds prior to her surgery, she no longer sees that same chubby child with the flat chest when she looks in the mirror. Gay attributes her satisfaction to having realistic expectations going into the procedure.

"There are so many things in your life that you have no control over and that make you unhappy," she says. "If you are willing to tolerate the pain, here is something you can actually do to make you feel better about yourself, to take charge of your body and your life. You get used to your body after forty-four years. It is amazing to wake up one day and have an amazing body."

NAME: Elizabeth
PROCEDURE: Breast augmentation with a lift
BRA SIZE BEFORE: 34 A
BRA SIZE AFTER: 36 C
AGE WHEN SURGERY PERFORMED: 33
CURRENT AGE: 34
MARITAL STATUS: Married (engaged at the time of the surgery)
OCCUPATION: Self-employed graphic designer
HIGHEST LEVEL OF EDUCATION: High school graduate, some
postgraduate study
NUMBER OF CHILDREN AND CURRENT AGES: Currently 13 weeks
pregnant

When asked why she had her surgery performed, Elizabeth emphasized that it was not to gain self-esteem, as this was something she already possessed. Rather, she did it because every time she went out she felt that she had to "booby trap" her bra to make it look like she had something in there. She was therefore limited in what she could wear and disliked that her bra size dictated her wardrobe. Although this was a longstanding issue with her, she had never really considered surgery previously. What finally triggered her decision was the purchase of her wedding dress. When looking at her gown, she commented to her fiancé, "This would look really great if I had breasts," to which he responded, "So go get the boobs." Although she had surgery for herself only, it was important to her that her fiancé was in favor of it.

Elizabeth became reluctant to undergo the procedure after seeing Dr. Freund, as she was informed that in her specific case it would not be as simple as slipping in a couple of implants, and that additional procedures and risks would be necessary. To Elizabeth, this was a real eye-opener and somewhat disappointing. She thought about it for several months before making the ultimate decision to go through with the procedure.

Aside from being very swollen after her surgery, Elizabeth didn't feel self-conscious about her new breasts. Her sexuality and her libido continued to be "great," and her partner's reaction was very positive. Although she did not feel uncomfortable when he touched her breasts, they did remain numb for six months due to her long healing process. Her friends were all thrilled and couldn't believe there were no scars, and some even hope to fix their sagging breasts.

When it came to confiding in her mother, who is a born-again Christian, Elizabeth elected to wait until a few months after the surgery was performed. She basically wanted to avoid any negative comments her mother might make until after she saw the final product. After seeing Elizabeth's new breasts, however, her mother was surprisingly ecstatic.

Elizabeth says she would definitely undergo her procedure again and feels it has enhanced her self-image. She is satisfied with the fact that she now has cleavage and can fit into clothes much better than she used to. She reports no level of dissatisfaction and indicates that having her breasts altered hasn't dramatically changed her life or the way she dresses. She has noticed that she gets more positive attention from people in that she will often catch them staring at her chest if she wears something tight. These looks of admiration are enjoyable to her, as she knows that her doctor did a good job, just as she can recognize bad "boob jobs" in others.

The only negative incident that she can recall was while working with a client she had met before her wedding. She had hoped to do a graphic design job for him but he cancelled on her multiple times. She didn't understand why this was occurring so she finally confronted him, to which the videographer expressed that he wasn't taking her seriously and was unsure if it was because of her blond hair or her big boobs. This was the only time she was made aware that her physical appearance could be a potential issue and affect the way people perceived her. However, she coped with this by disregarding what was said and continuing to do her job. In addition, she reminded herself that the size of her boobs has nothing to do with her abilities so she did not even acknowledge this ignorant comment.

Besides that incident, Elizabeth says her appearance has not changed the way males have reacted to her. She is just as assertive as before her surgery, so it hasn't changed the way she is treated by men. Because she doesn't walk around like a "floozy," she isn't treated as one. She says that many women have always been "catty" towards her, but she feels that is due to her strong personality, not to her change in bra size. She has always gotten dirty looks from women and believes that before her surgery they may have been jealous because they thought she had a great body, whereas now they think she has a *really* great body.

Finally, Elizabeth commented that if you are having cosmetic breast surgery for yourself, and it's something you truly desire and you have the financial means, then do it. However, she was quick to caution that you should only do it if you already have self-esteem, as it won't automatically provide that. To improve your self-esteem you should see a psychiatrist.

Jennifer N. Duffy, PhD, is a clinical psychologist and motivational corporate speaker who has appeared as a psychological consultant on many television talk shows, including *The Montel Williams Show, Ricki Lake,* and *Good Day New York.* She lives in Long Island, New York.

Taking Control of Your Recovery

Maximize Your Results with Vitamins, Supplements and Good Behavior

ONE OF THE THINGS that I like least about air travel is the fact that I have no control of the plane. My fate is in the hands of the pilot. Since I don't have a pilot's license or any experience whatsoever in the cockpit of an aircraft, I am completely dependent on the decisions being made by the person in the front seat.

Likewise, when you enter the realm of surgery, you are completely dependent upon the skill, knowledge, and good judgment of your surgeon and the surgical team. However, if you are well-informed (and if you are reading this book, you are!), there are many things that you can do to help your surgeon give you excellent results. Even while you are sleeping under anesthesia, the foods you ate, the medications you took, and your lifestyle in the weeks prior to your surgery can have a strong effect on how things go. And even more so, after you come out of surgery and embark on your road to recovery, though your doctor will still make recommendations and manage your recovery, there are many things that you can do to improve your results, speed your healing, and avoid complications. After all, your doctor will not live with you after your surgery. In fact, there will be a very limited number of hours that your doctor will be spending with you in the weeks following your surgery. What you do with those many hours when not with your doctor is very important to your recovery. So take control of your recovery! Do everything you can to help yourself achieve the best and most beautiful outcome for your breasts.

HERBAL SUPPLEMENTS

IN ASIA AND EUROPE, herbal remedies and traditional medicines are far more common than in the United States. But in the last several years, herbal supplements have become increasingly popular among patients. However, because these herbal supplements are not quite as popular with doctors as they are with patients, this has become a huge area of potential danger. Why a danger? Because most herbal supplements contain chemicals that enter the bloodstream, some of which may interact badly with prescription medications given to you by your doctor or may have negative effects on surgery. Because medical school does not train doctors on the subject of herbal and traditional medicines, many doctors are unaware of the potentially dangerous interactions and effects.

I will discuss a few of the currently known effects that some of the most popular herbal supplements may have on your surgery, both positive and negative. If you are taking any kind of homeopathic or herbal remedy that I don't cover here, you should certainly ask your doctor about it. If your doctor isn't sure, you should absolutely stop taking the supplement at least two weeks prior to surgery, and for at least two months following surgery. Because of the very real potential for problems, it's clearly better to be safe than sorry, and you can always resume taking the supplement after your recovery is complete.

For at least two weeks prior to surgery, you should avoid any supplements or homeopathic remedies that contain garlic, ginkgo biloba, ginger, Asian ginseng, or feverfew. All of these herbs slow blood coagulation by inhibiting the activity of platelets. This can delay healing, and, more seriously, can lead to excessive bleeding during surgery. The reaction can be more serious and dangerous if these herbs are used in conjunction with each other or with certain drugs that your doctor may administer during surgery. Some other herbs to watch out for are St. John's wort, kava, Echinacea, melatonin, and aloe vera, all of which affect the skin and could potentially have an adverse reaction on the healing of your scar.

However, not all herbs are harmful. One herbal supplement that is growing in popularity for patients recovering from plastic surgery is **arnica montana**. Some recent studies have indicated that arnica is not helpful in any meaningful way, but many patients and doctors swear by its effectiveness. The good news is that there seem to be no problematic side effects associated with arnica, and no reactions have ever been reported between arnica and the pre- and postoperative medications administered by surgeons. In other words, there is no downside to taking arnica. The companies selling arnica claim that taking it reduces swelling and bruising and aides in healing after surgery. The jury is still out on whether or not it works, but certainly there is no harm in taking this supplement if you want to give it a try.

Another herb, allium cepa, an onion extract that is sold under the brand name Mederma, is also gaining popularity. Mederma is a gel that is applied directly to the scar to speed healing and reduce scarring. Like arnica, there are conflicting studies as to how effective Mederma is. But, like arnica, there is no strong reason not to try this treatment.

After your scar is completely healed, rose hip oil is an herbal remedy that has been effective in reducing the appearance of the scar if used consistently for several months. Rose hip oil contains many important fatty acids that help the body repair skin and damaged tissues, and it has been found somewhat effective in reducing the color and appearance of scars.

As for other herbs and traditional medicines not covered here, I will again stress that when in doubt, cut it out. For at least two weeks prior to your surgery and for two months following, do not use any herbal supplements not specifically recommended by your doctor.

NUTRITION AND OVER-THE-COUNTER MEDICATIONS

BEYOND HERBAL REMEDIES, many vitamins, minerals, and over-the-counter medications also play important roles in your body's ability to cope effectively with surgery. Pain medications, in particular, can present a danger to your surgery, since most of them inhibit blood clotting and can lead to excessive bleeding during surgery. For a headache or muscle pain in the two weeks prior to your surgery, acetaminophen (Tylenol) is the only medication you should use unless specifically directed by your doctor. All others, including aspirin, Advil, Aleve, Anacin, Bufferin, Excedrin, ibuprofen, Motrin, naproxen sodium, and Naprosyn, as well as the prescription analgesics, Ketoralac and Toradol, should be avoided. MAO inhibitors, like Nardil and Parnate, should also be avoided for at least four weeks prior to surgery. If you are taking any of these medications (see pages 184–185 for a complete list), you should discuss alternatives with your doctor.

Vitamins and minerals also can have significant effects on healing. Nutrition is extremely important prior to surgery. For a month before your surgery you should eat well. Extra protein in your diet is a good idea to support healing both before and after surgery. Additionally, taking a multivitamin every day for a month is also a good idea to supplement vitamins and minerals, especially A and zinc, which are essential to healing. I recommend that all of my patients take 1,000 milligrams of vitamin ester C for a full month prior to surgery and for two months following surgery. Vitamin C is crucial to your body's ability to build strong collagen and for wound healing. During the course of wound healing, your body will use up much more vitamin C than normal. I recommend that you find a vitamin C in "ester" form (read the label on the bottle) because it is more easily absorbed by the body. Lastly, vitamin K is essential to healing and proper blood clotting associated with surgery. I give my patients a prescription strength version of vitamin K called Mephyton and have them begin taking it two days before surgery. You should request a prescription of Mephyton from your doctor if one was not already provided.

The one fact about vitamins that most of my patient's find surprising is that it is important not to take vitamin E for two weeks before your surgery. Many sources tout the usefulness of vitamin E oil in minimizing scars, but, in fact, because vitamin E prevents collagen-cross linkage, it tends to actually make scars wider. Avoid taking vitamin E supplements before your surgery and do not apply vitamin E to your scar for at least a few months after surgery.

The last point on nutrition is that you should avoid spicy or salty foods for a few days before and a week after surgery. While no extensive studies have been done on the subject, there is some evidence that these foods increase swelling and inflammation.

FURTHER PRODUCTS TO CONSIDER

A FEW OTHER products you should be aware of can help you take control of your recovery after your surgery. The first is **silicone sheeting** and silicone gels. Your surgeon will almost certainly discuss these products with you. Silicone sheeting is probably the most effective remedy for minimizing scars. The silicone sheeting is cut to size and must be held against the scar area with tape or bandages and should be worn as close to twenty-four hours a day as possible. Once a day the sheet should be removed, washed with mild soap, and replaced. For some incision sites silicone sheeting might be too difficult to use properly. In these cases, the second best alternative is silicone gel. The gel is applied over the incision area and it dries to a similar consistency as the sheeting.

Silicone products are available in your pharmacy or from your surgeon, but be aware that not all silicone sheets are the same. One product, Rejuveness, is available at most pharmacies and may help flatten a scar but does not have the moisturizing effects of other more gelatinous types of silicone sheets, such as Novagel. Novagel is my first choice and is available in your surgeon's office.

Neosporin, a common antibacterial ointment, is supposed to improve the appearance of scars if used during the healing process. Some doctors recommend against it before the wound is fully closed, but it can be an effective way to keep the incision area soft during healing. Bacitracin, another common antibacterial ointment, should be avoided because of frequent problems with allergic reactions.

Another product on the market that is becoming increasingly popular is ScarGuard. ScarGuard, made by Byron Medical, combines several ingredients known to help in scar healing in one quick-drying liquid. It may be a very effective medication for reducing scars; however, it important not to use ScarGuard early on in the healing process because it contains vitamin E and may tend to slow healing and actually create a wider scar than is necessary.

To help you make sense of all this information, you can review all of the above in the quick reference table below.

GUIDE TO VITAMINS, MINERALS, AND OVER-THE-COUNTER MEDICATIONS

PRODUCT NAME	BEFORE SURGERY	AFTER SURGERY
Aloe Vera	No	No
Arnica Montana	Yes	Yes
Acetominophen	Okay	Okay
Advil	No	No
Aleve	No	No
Anacin	No	No
Aspirin	No	No
Bacitracin	No	No
Bufferin	No	No
Echinacea	No	No
Excedrin	No	No
Feverfew	No	No
Garlic supplements	No	No
Ginger	No	No
Ginseng (Asian)	No	No
Ginko biloba	No	No
Ibuprofen	No	No
Kava	No	No
Ketoralac	No	No
MAO Inhibitors	No	No
Mederma	No	After healing
Melatonin	No	No

PRODUCT NAME	BEFORE SURGERY	AFTER SURGERY
Motrin	No	No
Naprosyn	No	No
Naproxin Na	No	No
Nardil	No	No
Neosporin	No	Okay
Parnate	No	No
Rose hip oil	No	After healing
ScarGuard	No	After healing
Silicone gel	No	Yes
Silicone sheeting	No	Yes
Spicy foods	No, 2 days	No, 1 week
St. John's wort	No	No
Toradol	No	No
Tylenol	Okay	Okay
Vitamin A	In multivitamin	In multivitamin
Vitamin C	1000 mg, 4 weeks	1000 mg, 8 weeks
Vitamin E	No	No
Vitamin K (Mephyton)	2 days	1 week
Zinc	In multivitamin	In multivitamin

FURTHER WAYS TO TAKE CONTROL OF YOUR HEALING PROCESS

ONE THING THAT many patients have found very helpful is to keep a list of questions. You should begin your list even before your first consultation with your surgeon. Keep your list somewhere convenient—on a bulletin board that you use frequently, on your refrigerator, on top of your desk at work, or on the nightstand by your bed. The important thing is that you can immediately write down any question as soon as it arises in your mind. Take your list with you whenever you have an appointment with your doctor and make sure that every question that you have is answered and that you fully understand the answer *before* your surgery. Not only will this ensure that you have all of the necessary information prior to surgery, but also it is important for your mental state to not have any nagging doubts when you go into surgery. A good attitude is important for good healing.

Another thing to keep in mind in the weeks before your surgery is that you don't want to have any stressful or difficult things to do in the early weeks of your recovery. You should make every effort to leave nothing to chance for those weeks. Everything should be done as early as possible before your surgery. This may include things like arranging for child care, making sure that everything—from taking time off from work to organizing the things that need to be done in your household—are taken care of or arranged for. Nobody at work should need to call you for any emergencies when you're busy healing. Certainly you want to make sure that you've prepared everything in your home for easy access. Anything that's on a high shelf that you think you might want access to in those first few weeks of recovery should be taken down and put within easy reach without lifting your arms. All of the prescriptions that your doctor gives you for after your surgery must be filled before your surgery. Make sure all of your arrangements for getting to and from the hospital or office are taken care of and confirmed. You will need someone reliable to escort you home.

Another thing to take care of is purchasing two new bras to be worn after your surgery. Your doctor will give you some recommendations in this area because different procedures will require different types of bras, but there are a few simple guidelines. Most importantly, the bras you purchase must fasten in the front. You can forget reaching behind you or pulling them over your head in the first few days after your operation. For enlargements and lifts you'll need sports bras, preferably with a zipper in the front. Breast reduction bras should not have underwires.

PREPARING FOR YOUR SURGERY

IF YOU'VE DONE a good job and taken care of all of these things early, you'll be able to concentrate on the small list of things to remember the night before and the day of your surgery. Refer to "Your Pre- and Post-Surgery Checklist" at the back of this book for a complete list of things to remember. Make sure you don't eat or drink anything after midnight the day of your operation. It's easy to forget and get a glass of water in the night. Take your supplements, vitamin C, or Mephyton before midnight because you won't be taking them the day of your surgery.

The morning of your surgery there are a few things to keep in mind. Make sure you wear very comfortable, loose clothing that zippers or buttons in the front. Putting clothing back on that slips over the head might be impossible after your operation. Sweats or drawstring pants are preferred. No jeans. Clothing in dark colors is a good idea since there may be a bit of bleeding. You may be a little dizzy after surgery from the anesthesia and you should only wear flat shoes or sneakers. It is very important to wear absolutely no makeup or moisturizers anywhere on your body. Many cosmetics contain traces of metallic chemicals that can interfere with some of the electronic equipment used in modern surgery. Leave it off. Naturally, this also means absolutely no jewelry anywhere. Remove all piercings from every part of the body, from the eyebrows to the toes, and leave them at home.

You are ready!

Your doctor will probably have given you a prescription for Zofran. This is an anti-nausea medication that you may need after your surgery because some people become nauseous from the pain medication. Two hours before your surgery you should take one Zofran with a tiny sip of water. This will help keep you from becoming nauseous from the anesthesia when you wake in the recovery area.

AFTER YOUR SURGERY

WHEN YOUR SURGERY is over, the surgeon's job is largely over. You'll still have doctor appointments for him or her to check on your healing and later to remove stitches and other small items of this nature, but most of the doctor's work happens in the operating room. Now it's largely up to you.

Your first priority should be to follow all of your doctor's instructions as closely as possible. It is very possible that you will feel far better than expected. You may feel that because you are recovering quickly that you can begin activities, such as sleeping on your stomach or not wearing your bra constantly sooner than recommended by your doctor. Forget about it! Do everything right and you won't have any regrets later. Waiting a few more days before exercise won't hurt you; putting stress on your surgery earlier than recommended might.

You should leave your surgical tape on for as long as possible, or at least as long as your doctor recommends. The tape placed over the wounds after your surgery is designed to keep weight, tension, and stress off of the healing incision site. This is one of the best ways to help maintain even healing and have nice, clean, minimal scars.

Depending upon your surgery, you may experience quite a bit of pain in the first few days after your procedure. Your doctor will have given you a prescription for a painkiller, probably a narcotic such as Vicodin or Percocet. Both of these medications are very effective, but can be addictive if you use them too frequently and for too long. This should not be a problem if you use them only as needed and not on a schedule. Another possible problem with narcotics in general is nausea. Not all women will have this problem, but if it does become an issue, the Zofran should help. Like Vicodin, Zofran should only be used as needed. One frustration associated with the nausea caused by Vicodin (for patients who experience it) is that the analgesic effect of the medication only works for about three to four hours, but the nausea generally persists for up to eight hours. Constipation is also a common problem associated with Vicodin. Just a few more reasons to only use it as necessary.

Your doctor will have also given you prescriptions for antibiotics. Unlike the painkillers, you must take your antibiotics on schedule and finish every pill prescribed. Regardless of how well you feel or any other factors, it is very important to be extremely diligent with your antibiotics. Take every pill on schedule and finish them on schedule.

Depending on the type of surgery performed, you may be able to start showering on the second day after surgery. Of course, every physician has his own routine, and you should strictly adhere to your doctor's advice. Be careful to keep water from spraying directly on the dressings. After showering, pat the dressings dry, and apply some dry gauze. You want these dressings to stay as clean, dry, and intact as possible.

Wear your bra. It is important to wear a bra as much as possible, day and night, for six weeks after surgery.

You should be able to resume light exercise after three weeks, provided you are careful and that you don't do anything that requires you to use your upper body. Walking or riding a stationary bicycle are two good options. Riding a real bicycle outside is a bad idea because you may have to put weight on the handlebars, and, more significantly, any kind of accident could have catastrophic results for your surgery. After six weeks you should feel comfortable to begin light exercise with your upper body.

All of the suggestions in this chapter may seem like a great many things to do and to keep track of, but, taken together they can be a very effective way for you to contribute to your success and get the best possible results. Cosmetic breast surgery is a big decision and you will live with the results for many, many years. You will spend a great deal of money on the process. You will spend time and deal with pain and inconvenience. You owe it to yourself to take control of your recovery and to do everything possible to get the outcome that you desire.

Teens and Cosmetic Breast Surgery

Guidance for Parents in the Age of Britney and Christina

MORE AND MORE frequently I am asked about teens and cosmetic breast surgery. Currently, there is so much in the media regarding teen body image and speculation about teen stars, like Britney Spears and Christina Aguilera, having breast augmentation before their eighteenth birthdays seems to be everywhere. And, of course, in Hollywood, teen bodies with perfect breasts are everywhere.

To begin this discussion in the correct manner, it is important to state that it is illegal to perform cosmetic breast surgery on girls under the age of eighteen. Exceptions can be made, particularly in the case of breast reductions for reasons of health and medical necessity. Certainly it is always illegal and certainly unwise to do breast implant surgery on a very young teen except in the case of reconstruction following cancer or a disfiguring injury.

Breast reduction in boys suffering from **gynecomastia** and girls who are suffering from some sort of debilitation due to breast size, such as back and neck pain, skin rashes, and shoulder grooving, can be considered "reconstructive," rather than cosmetic and will usually be covered by insurance companies. They may also cover the correction of very asymmetrical breasts. Even in these cases, it may be necessary to wait if the surgeon believes that the normal growth cycle is not completed. If the procedure is done and the breasts continue to grow, this may create abnormalities, and it may be more difficult or even impossible to do a second surgery after normal growth is completed due to compromised blood supply.

For girls who are still growing but are already suffering from negative symptoms due to excessive breast size, one stopgap measure may be the use of liposuction. While liposuction is very unlikely to completely solve the problem, it may offer enough relief in the short term to allow the teen to wait until her growth cycle is complete before having her breast reduction surgery.

GUIDELINES FOR PARENTS

THE EMOTIONAL MATURITY of teens can make decisions about cosmetic surgery far more complicated. The American Society for Aesthetic Plastic Surgery offers parents some guidelines that may also be useful.

First, parents should never suggest plastic surgery to a teen. If the teen brings it up, a parent should feel free to discuss the option at length, but it is very inadvisable and potentially quite damaging to a teen's self-esteem for the parent to suggest the idea first. In some cases where the parent suspects that the teen is thinking about or even talking about plastic surgery with friends but is too embarrassed to discuss it with the parent, it may be possible to ask some open-ended questions that will make the teen feel more comfortable in raising the question.

Parents need to be especially careful about unrealistic ideas that teens have about plastic surgery and how it will change their lives. Often a teen's desire for plastic surgery will have more to do with a problem of ego than a problem of breast size. Teens who believe that different breasts will make them more popular probably need something that plastic surgery will be unable to offer them. You should have a very frank discussion with your teen about why she wants cosmetic breast surgery, what she thinks the problem with her breasts is, how long it has bothered her, and how she thinks it will change her life to have the problem corrected. This will allow you to assess how realistic her feelings and goals are for plastic surgery.

Finally, parents must consider the teen's emotional maturity. They should remember that during the teen years there is a powerful desire among teens to be like their peers. Individuality is less accepted until later adolescence. If this seems to be a driving force behind your teen's desire for cosmetic breast surgery you should be very cautious of her very real emotional turmoil and be respectful of her feelings. It is also important to assess if your teen has the maturity to deal with the pain and temporary physical disfigurement that the surgery will involve. Teens that are dealing with other emotional issues such as depression or drug addiction are probably poor candidates for cosmetic breast surgery.

If your teen's feelings regarding cosmetic breast surgery are repeated frequently and in realistic terms, it may be something that you should consider. Consulting a plastic surgeon at this time can be very helpful. The surgeon can do a professional assessment of the teen's physical and emotional maturity and give your teen important and realistic information regarding what can and can't be accomplished through plastic surgery. It is a very good idea to allow the surgeon to consult with the teen alone, outside of your presence. Most teens will speak more freely about embarrassing issues outside of their parent's presence—especially with a doctor, who is neither peer nor part of the teen's social world. Additionally, many teens feel different kinds of parental pressure, whether realistic or not, that will inhibit frank discussion.

If a teen is constantly talking about seeking cosmetic breast surgery, another consideration might be Body Dysmorphic Disorder or BDD. Experts believe that as many as five million people suffer from BDD in the United States and the most common time for onset of this condition is, not surprisingly, during adolescence. BDD is characterized by obsessive dissatisfaction with a particular body part. The person suffering from BDD may hate his or her nose or their legs or their hips, but it is not uncommon for adolescent girls to focus their dysphoria on their breasts.

A girl who has BDD may or may not have anything at all wrong with her breasts. A slight asymmetry or even a completely imagined flaw may completely absorb her attention. In clinical research on BDD, women who had these negative feelings about their breasts often became obsessed with the idea of plastic surgery as a solution—however, in almost all of these cases, regardless of the procedure and its level of success, cosmetic surgery did nothing to improve their satisfaction with their breasts. Needless to say, patients who suffer from BDD are something of a nightmare for cosmetic surgeons who, as a rule, crave the delight of their patients for their own professional satisfaction!

In extreme cases, BDD can ruin lives. How do you know if your teen is suffering from BDD and not just a rational dissatisfaction with her breasts? People who suffer from BDD are not only obsessed with the body part in question, but they have an irrational belief that everybody else is obsessed with it also. If your daughter is unhappy and overly preoccupied with her breasts, and firmly believes that people don't like her or shun her as a friend because of her breasts, perhaps a cosmetic surgeon is not the kind of doctor that you should be seeking.

IT'S GOOD TO WAIT

DEALING WITH A TEEN who is unhappy with her body is never an easy proposition and it seems to be an ever more common problem in our society. Even a cosmetic surgeon, who makes his or her living helping people change their bodies, must ultimately realize that it is unhealthy for a society to overemphasize the importance of how people look. The laws that protect teens from undergoing procedures like breast augmentation before they are eighteen are very appropriate. For teens that are teased because of their breasts or embarrassed in the locker room, there may be some temptation on the part of the parents or the surgeon to convince the lawmakers or the insurance companies that there is a "medical necessity" for the surgery. People will be embarrassed and teased over many things— especially during their teen years, but also throughout their lives. Learning to live with a problem as small as physical appearance is a life lesson worth learning. Even the most mature and level-headed teen will not suffer greatly if she is forced to wait until her eighteenth birthday before having cosmetic breast surgery. Furthermore, she will have that surgery with the benefit of greater maturity and a greater appreciation for others who are not physically perfect.

Your Pre- and Post-Surgery Checklist

▷ Within 30 days prior to surgery

❑ **Ask questions.** Although you have gotten past the biggest decision and confidently chosen to have surgery, the reality of the situation almost always generates many more questions. Write down all of your questions and concerns and relay them to your surgeon. The responses will typically allay your fears and strengthen the relationship between you and your surgeon.

❑ **Get tested.** Have all pre-surgical testing (blood tests, mammograms, medical clearance examinations) performed according to your physician's requirements. Make sure all results are relayed to your surgeon's office.

❑ **Stop smoking.** Enough said.

❑ **DON'T take** aspirin and vitamin E, which can interfere with the surgery.*

❏ **DO take** vitamin Ester C and a multivitamin to help your body prepare for your surgery. Take Tylenol only for pain.*

❏ **Discuss** all medications, vitamins, minerals, and herbal supplements with your physician. Many supplements may interfere with blood clotting during surgery.*

▷ 14 Days prior to surgery

❏ **Visit the pharmacy.** Fill all of your prescriptions as provided by your surgeon and get a layman's description of each medication's purpose, as well as an explanation of when to take each one.

❏ **Find a post-surgery helper.** Arrange for someone to escort you home after surgery and care for you in the post-operative period. Each procedure is different, and each woman's post-surgical experience is different. Get an idea from your physician as to the length of time you will be out of commission.

❏ **Buy bras.** You will need to buy two new bras to be worn after your surgery. Consult your physician as to the type of bra necessary for your particular procedure, as different procedures will require different types of bras. I generally recommend front-fastening bras (with a zipper or hooks) and sports bras for all breast lifts and enlargements. Breast reduction bras should not have underwires.

▷ 2 Days prior to surgery

❏ **Call** your surgeon's office to confirm surgery time.

❑ **Watch what you eat.** Avoid salty or spicy foods from now until one week after surgery.

▷ The night before surgery

❑ **Fast.** Do not eat or drink *anything* after midnight the night prior to surgery.

❑ **Talk to your anesthesiologist.** For in-office procedures, it is routine for the anesthesiologist to call you the night before surgery to review your history and answer any questions you may have regarding anesthesia.

▷ The day of surgery

❑ **Dress comfortably.** Wear loose fitting clothing: a zipper or button down shirt and drawstring or slip-on pants (no jeans). Wear flat shoes or sneakers.

❑ **Do not wear** any make-up, moisturizers, lotion, deodorant or contact lenses.

❑ **Leave** jewelry (including any body piercings) and valuables at home.

❑ **Bring** all of your medications with you.

▷ After surgery

❑ **Expect discomfort.** You may experience pain or pressure. This is normal and should be relieved by the medications prescribed. If you do not get relief, or the pain worsens, call your doctor.

❑ **Sleep on your back.** Do not lie on your side or stomach for six weeks.

❑ **Hygiene.** When to shower and exercise depends on your procedure. Consult with your physician to get clear instructions regarding these activities.

❑ **Don't panic.** Your breasts will get smaller and change shape for up to six months after surgery as a result of swelling. Do not get upset or overly concerned if they appear larger than desired in the early post-operative period. However, if one or both breasts become large, hard, and acutely very painful after surgery, this may be a sign that bleeding has occurred around the implants and you should call your surgeon to discuss these issues.

❑ **Don't take** aspirin or vitamin E for 10 days after surgery.*

* See pages 184–185 for a guide to vitamins, minerals, and over-the-counter medications.

Glossary

AAAASF. American Association for the Accreditation of Ambulatory Surgery Facilities. A physician-run association set up to establish standards and ensure compliance of these standards in ambulatory surgical facilities.

AAHC. American Accreditation Healthcare Commission—formerly known as Utilization Review Accreditation Commission. Performs evaluation and utilization of ambulatory care facilities.

ACCOLATE. A prescription medication for asthma that has been shown to reduce the severity of capsular contracture in some patients.

AMERICAN BOARD OF PLASTIC SURGERY. The governing board that certifies all plastic surgeons. This is the only board that certifies plastic surgeons.

ANATOMICAL IMPLANT. Breast implants uniquely shaped to provide a more natural breast shape by altering their height or width.

ANESTHESIA. Drugs and gases designed to eliminate pain and awareness of the ongoing surgery.

AREOLA. The pigmented area surrounding the nipple.

ARNICA MONTANA. An herbal supplement that is touted to reduce bruising and swelling. There is no scientific evidence to support these claims.

ASPIRATE. A technique for removal of hematoma or seroma by using a thin needle-like instrument.

ASYMMETRY. When two breasts are unequal in shape, size, or nipple position.

AUGMENTATION. Another term used for enlargement. In the case of this book, used to indicate breast enlargement with implants.

AUTOIMMUNE DISEASES. A group of diseases related to the patient's own immune system. The immune system reacts against the patient's own tissues causing organ malfunction.

AXILLARY TECHNIQUE. See *trans-axillary technique*.

BAKER SCALE. A measurement of the advancement of capsular contracture based upon subjective factors, such as the appearance and feel of the breasts.

BODY DYSMORPHIC DISORDER. The irrational dissatisfaction with a part of one's own body.

BRAVA. A proprietary device designed to enlarge breasts by applying a vacuum suction to the breasts.

BREAD-LOAFING. See Symmastia.

BREAST PROJECTION. A descriptive term to explain the amount of breast tissue that protrudes forward on the chest wall.

CAPSULAR CONTRACTURE. When the normal capsule that the body forms around any foreign object begins to contract around a breast implant, potentially causing complications.

CAPSULECTOMY. The surgical removal of the capsule that forms around an implant due to advanced capsular contracture.

CAPSULOTOMY. The breaking of the capsule that forms around an implant in order to relieve the pressure caused by capsular contracture. Also see *Closed capsulotomy*.

CC. Cubic centimeter. A measure of volume equivalent to a milliliter.

CHEST WALL. The tissue, cartilage, and bone (ribs) of the chest that sit beneath the muscle and gland tissue of the breast.

CIRCUMAREOLAR INCISION. A surgical incision made around the areola, the colored area around the nipple.

CLOSED CAPSULOTOMY. The breaking of the capsule formed around an implant by squeezing the breast between the hands. This procedure is not recommended.

CONTACT INHIBITION. The cellular process that tells cells to stop multiplying when they come into contact with each other.

DIEP FLAP PROCEDURE. DIEP stands for Deep Inferior Epigastric Perforator. A breast reconstruction technique similar to the TRAM flap technique but which attempts to spare the abdominal muscles that are weakened in the normal TRAM flap procedure. It is not recommended at the time of writing.

DOUBLE BUBBLE. A transverse crease on the lower half of the breast skin after breast augmentation.

EKLUND TECHNIQUE. The series of X-ray views for effectively taking mammograms with implants. Two extra views are required, which could mean additional exposure to X-ray radiation.

ENDOSCOPE. A flexible tube with a camera mounted on the end for performing remote surgery.

EXPANDER. See *Tissue expander*.

FREE-NIPPLE PROCEDURE. A type of breast reduction procedure for very large breasts in which the nipple-areolar complex is removed from the breast tissue and replaced as a graft. As a result, the patient's ability to breast-feed or become stimulated will be lost.

GOËS TECHNIQUE. A technique for small breast reduction or breast lifts with the scar only around the areola.

GOULIAN MASTOPEXY. A breast lift which leaves an anchor-shaped scar.

GYNECOMASTIA. A medical condition that causes the appearance of female-like breasts in men.

HALL-FINDLAY TECHNIQUE. A modified version of the vertical scar technique for breast reduction. Similar to the Lejour technique.

HEMATOMA. A collection or pocket of blood within the tissue of the body.

HIGH PROFILE BREAST IMPLANT. A breast implant with a more narrow diameter designed to create added breast projection.

IMPLANT. A medical device made of either silicone or saline (saltwater), designed to add volume and shape to a woman's breasts.

IMPLANT PTOSIS. When a breast implant sags below the natural shape of the breast.

INFERIOR PEDICLE TECHNIQUE. A technique for large volume breast reduction that involves maintaining a flap of tissue beneath and including the nipple and requiring an anchor-shaped scar.

INFRAMAMMARY FOLD. The area on the underside of the breast where it attaches to the body.

INFRAMAMMARY TECHNIQUE. An augmentation technique in which the incision for breast augmentation is placed on or near the inframammary fold.

INTERNAL PHYSIOLOGIC BREAST SPLINT. A technique to raise the inframammary fold in patients with a low fold after previous breast augmentation surgery.

JCAHO. Joint Commission on Accreditation of Healthcare Organizations. An independent, private, non-profit organization that evaluates, sets standards for, and accredits hospitals and ambulatory care facilities.

KELOID SCAR. A scar that is raised, hard, and grows outside the original incision boundaries.

LATERAL CHEST BREAK. The distance that the breast extends outward to the side of the chest, giving rise to the top portion of the "hour-glass" figure.

LIPOSUCTION. A technique for removing fat by vacuum aspiration.

LEJOUR TECHNIQUE. A technique for breast lift or reduction that provides maximum breast projection and long-lasting results. It leaves a "lollipop"-shaped scar.

MAMMAPLASTY. Any plastic surgery to alter the size or shape of the breasts.

MAMMOGRAM. An X ray used to examine the female breast. Implants obscure visualization of some breast tissue, thereby limiting the benefit of mammograms.

MASTECTOMY. The surgical term for the removal of a breast.

MASTITIS. A breast infection.

MASTOPEXY. Any plastic surgery on the breasts in which the breast is lifted or reshaped.

MCKISSOCK TECHNIQUE. A technique for the reshaping and reduction of the breast that leaves an anchor-shaped scar.

MRI. A diagnostic study (radiation-free) that is excellent for examining soft tissue (including breast tissue). Implants do not obscure visualization of breast tissue in an MRI, so it is excellent for breast visualization in patients with implants.

NECROSIS. The death of a localized area of tissue or cells of the body.

NIPPLE-AREOLA COMPLEX. The part of the breast that includes the nipple and the surrounding darker skin.

"NO TOUCH TECHNIQUE." A technique for beast enlargement whereby the implants are transferred from the shipping package to the breast without being handled by the surgeon's gloves or coming in contact with the patient's skin. It is hypothesized that handling of the implants can contribute to an increase in implant capsular contracture.

PAIN PUMP. A device designed to slowly release pain medication to the site of operation.

PARENCHYMA. Soft organ or gland tissue.

PECTORAL MUSCLES. The large muscles of the chest that lie beneath the breast.

PECTORAL SHELF DEFORMITY. A poor result from plastic surgery caused by a lack of tissue at the top of the breast and characterized by the abrupt protrusion of the implant from the center of the chest, resulting in a "shelf-like" appearance.

PEDICLE FLAP. The portion of a tissue graft that is left attached to the underlying tissue and blood supply.

PERIAREOLAR TECHNIQUE. An incision site that runs along the bottom rim of the areola.

POLAND'S SYNDROME. A syndrome that creates a deficiency of the breast, pectoralis major, and minor muscles, as well as the arm on the affected side.

POSTOPERATIVELY ADJUSTABLE IMPLANT. An implant with an accessory port for adjusting the size after surgery. The port is removed after adjustments are completed.

PSEUDOPTOSIS. The condition where the breasts are sagging but the nipple remains in a normal position. Also called "Bottoming out."

PTOSIS. A technical term for sagging of the breasts.

PURSE-STRING STITCHING TECHNIQUE. The surgical technique whereby a large circle is reduced to a smaller size. Typically used during circumareolar breast reductions and lifts.

RICE TEST. An at-home test that allows patients to test for the proper implant size. Rice is portioned in a measuring cup, and then transferred to a plastic bag or panty hose. The rice is then inserted into the patient's bra to simulate the actual breast enlargement.

ROTATION FLAP PROCEDURE. A technique whereby tissue is taken from one anatomic position and rotated into another position.

SEROMA. Similar to a *hematoma*. A collection or pocket of clear fluid within the body.

SERUM. A component of blood that leaks into wounds after surgery or trauma.

SILICONE. A polymer or complex molecule that is based on the element silicon.

SILICONE GEL. A gelatinous substance made of silicone. The gel is used for filing silicone gel implants. It had been found to be helpful in reducing scarring and redress when applied topically to a healing scar.

SILICONE SHEETING. A sheet of silicone that is applied externally to a healing incision to minimize scarring and redness.

SUBGLANDULAR. A placement site for breast implants that lies above the muscle and below the gland of the breast.

SUBMUSCULAR. A placement site for breast implants that lies beneath most of the pectoral muscle.

SYMMASTIA. Also called bread-loafing. A complication in breast augmentation surgery where the implants migrate together giving the appearance of a single breast in the middle of the chest.

TEARDROP AUGMENTATION MASTOPEXY. A breast lift/enlargement technique that lifts and shapes breast tissue from above and below the breast tissue, creating a teardrop-shaped breast with added durability.

TISSUE EXPANDER. A balloon-like device for gradually increasing the size of the pocket inside the muscle or breast tissue before insertion of an implant.

TOXIC SHOCK SYNDROME (TSS). An acute infection of the blood as a result of bacterial contamination that leads to failure of multiple organs. In rare occurrences it can be associated with an infected breast implant.

TRAM FLAP. The Transverse Rectus Abdominus Myocutaneous flap—the muscle and overlaying skin of the lower abdomen that is frequently used as a tissue donor site for breast reconstruction following mastectomy.

TRANS-AXILLARY TECHNIQUE. The technique for inserting a breast implant using an endoscope through the armpit.

TRANS-UMBILICAL ENDOSCOPIC AUGMENTATION (TUBA) TECHNIQUE. The technique for inserting a breast implant using an endoscope through the belly button. This technique is not recommended.

TUBULAR BREASTS. Breasts with wide, ballooning nipple-areola complexes, narrow bases to the breasts, and tube-like shapes.

VERTICAL SCAR BREAST REDUCTION. See *Lejour technique.*

WISE PATTERN. See *McKissock technique.*

Internet Resources

WWW.INAMED.COM The parent company of McGhan implants provides a fair and balanced website that offers large amounts of information about breast implants as well as their risks. At the current time, McGhan is the only company approved to provide silicone implants to most patients.

WWW.MENTORCORP.COM Mentor Company is the second largest implant company in the United States. This website also offers a fair and balanced view of implant surgery.

WWW.BREASTCANCERCARE.ORG A well-organized site that will explain all facets of breast cancer, treatments, reconstructive options, and associated treatments, like chemotherapy and radiation

WWW.BREASTHEALTHONLINE.ORG A global nonprofit organization dedicated to providing information and support for women going through breast augmentation, breast reduction, and breast reconstruction.

WWW.SURGERY.ORG A website for the American Society for Aesthetic Plastic Surgery. This site provides information about a wide range of cosmetic surgery topics and lists all members of its organization in referral form. As always, do your homework on all referrals.

WWW.PLASTICSURGERY.ORG Website for the American Society of Plastic Surgeons. This site is similar to the previous site, offering news and information on a wide array of plastic surgical techniques.

WWW.ABMS.ORG A website hosted by the American Board of Medical Specialties. This site will help you examine your physicians' board certifications. It also explains the importance of board certification and the requirements met by your physician to become certified.

Acknowledgments

THANK YOU TO my family: my wife Judy, Jake, Ben, and Emily for their encouragement and loving support. Thank you to my staff: Paula, Aimee, Torrey, and Bibi for their technical assistance and encouragement. Finally, thanks to Nicolas Tabbal for being a true gentleman and wonderful role model.

Index

About the Authors

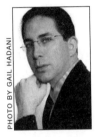

PHOTO BY GAIL HADANI

ROBERT M. FREUND, MD, FACS, is an innovative and highly sought-after plastic surgeon with his own private practice and privileges at New York City's Lenox Hill, Beth Israel, and Manhattan Eye, Ear, and Throat Hospitals. His state-of-the-art teardrop augmentation mastopexy has been accepted as the latest and most impressive improvement in cosmetic breast surgery. He has lectured all over the U.S. and abroad, and has appeared on NBC, Fox News, and in *Men's Health* magazine. He lives in Old Westbury, New York.

ALEXANDER VAN DYNE is a freelance screenwriter and novelist who has learned to translate the sometimes inscrutable language of doctors. He lives in New York City.